INTERNATIONAL PERSPECTIVES IN EXERCISE PHYSIOLOGY

Krystyna Nazar, MD
Polish Academy of Sciences

Ronald L. Terjung, PhD
State University of New York

Hanna Kaciuba-Uściłko, PhD
Leszek Budohoski, PhD
Polish Academy of Sciences

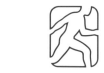

Human Kinetics Books
Champaign, Illinois

Library of Congress Cataloging-in-Publication Data

International perspectives in exercise physiology / editors, Krystyna
Nazar ... [et al.].
    p.   cm.
   Proceedings of the International Symposium on Exercise Physiology
in honor of Stanisław Kozłowski, held at Baranów Sandomierski,
Poland on June 18-20, 1987.
   Includes bibliographical references.
   ISBN 0-87322-283-0
   1. Exercise--Physiological aspects--Congresses. I. Nazar,
Krystyna, 1939-   . II. International Symposium on Exercise
Physiology (1987 : Baranów Sandomierski, Poland)
QP301.I56 1990   67671
612'.044--dc20   89-37079
                                                           CIP

ISBN: 0-87322-283-0

Proceedings of the International Symposium in Memory of Stanisław Kozłowski, held in
Baranów Sandomierski Castle, Poland, June 18-20, 1987.

Developmental Editor: Kathy Kane
Assistant Editor: Timothy Ryan
Copyeditor: Kathy Kane
Proofreader: Karin Leszczynski
Production Director: Ernie Noa
Typesetter: Brad Colson
Text Design: Keith Blomberg
Text Layout: Jill Wikgren
Cover Design: Carlson Communications
Printer: Braun-Brumfield, Inc.

Printed in the United States of America

10 9 8 7 6 5 4 3 2 1

Human Kinetics Books
A Division of Human Kinetics Publishers, Inc.
Box 5076, Champaign, IL 61825-5076
1-800-747-4HKP

INTERNATIONAL
PERSPECTIVES
IN EXERCISE
PHYSIOLOGY

Contents

Part II: *Exercise Metabolism and Performance*   61

Research Notes

Part III: *Energy Metabolism and Its Control* 103

Research Notes

Symposium Organization

This volume represents the Proceedings of the International Symposium on Exercise Physiology dedicated to the memory of the late Professor Stanisław Kozłowski, held at Baranów Sandomierski, Poland, June 18–20, 1987.

Medical Research Centre, Polish Academy of Sciences
Polish Society of Sports Medicine
Polish Physiological Society
Local Authorities of Tarnobrzeg Province

Organizing Committee

Honorary President: Professor Ernst Jokl
President: Professor Mirosław Mossakowski
Vice Presidents: Professor Hanna Kaciuba-Uśiłko
Dr. Witold Furgał
Secretary General: Professor Krystyna Nazar
Members: Dr. Leszek Budohoski, Barbara Modzelewska, Assoc. Professor Dr. Ewa Szczepańska-Sadowska, and Dr. Andrzej W. Ziemba

Preface

The International Symposium on Exercise Physiology held at Baranów Sandomierski, Poland on June 18–20, 1987 was devoted to the memory of the late Professor Stanisław Kozłowski, the much beloved leader of exercise physiologists in Poland. The symposium attracted many distinguished physiologists from all over the world who wished to pay tribute to their deceased colleague and friend. The program of the symposium was prepared by professor Kozłowski's erstwhile colleagues, led by Professors Mirosław Mossakowski, Hanna Kaciuba-Uściłko, and Krystyna Nazar. Among the participants at Baranów Sandomierski were speakers from the USA, England, Sweden, Denmark, France, Japan, the USSR, Czechoslovakia, and Germany, in addition to well known scientists from Poland. The papers are of high quality, offering an abundance of useful information from an international perspective. The major themes in the text are the following:

- The present state and perspectives of exercise physiology,
- Cardiovascular adjustments and adaptation to physical exercise,
- Exercise metabolism and performance,
- Energy metabolism and its control,
- Endocrine responses to exercise and environmental changes,
- Thermoregulation and body temperature responses to exercise,
- Clinical aspects of physical activity, and a
- Panel discussion on basic physiological factors determining endurance performance.

On behalf of the foreign participants in the symposium in memory of the late Professor Stanisław Kozłowski I convey to the Polish hosts our sincere thanks, combined with the expression of admiration for their scientific contributions in the field of exercise physiology and sports medicine.

> Professor Ernst Jokl,
> Honorary President
> of the International Symposium
> on Exercise Physiology

Acknowledgments

On behalf of the Organizing Committee we wish to express our gratitude to all contributors of the Symposium from many countries of the world. We would also like to thank the following people who devoted considerable time to preparing for this meeting: the staff of the Departments of Applied Physiology, M.R.C., Polish Academy of Sciences and Medical School in Warsaw, our colleagues from the Sports Medicine Clinic in Tarnobrzeg, Mr. Marek Indyk, M.S., the Vice-Director of the Sulphur Production Plants, and Mrs. Stanisława Bochniewicz, M.S., the custodian of the Baranów Sandomierski Castle, where the Symposium took place.

Special thanks go to Mrs. Jadwiga Kozłowska, M.S. and Miss Ewa Kozłowska, M.D., who not only honored the meeting with their presence but also helped in the preparation of this book. We also wish to acknowledge the financial support provided by the Polish Society of Sports Medicine, the Sulphur Production Plants "Siarkopol," the Corning Glass Work Company, the E. Jaeger GmbH Company, and the Trade Centre of Sciences Ltd., Polish Academy of Sciences.

Hanna Kaciuba-Uścilko
Krystyna Nazar
Leszek Budohoski

Opening Messages

Professor Stanisław Kozłowski:
His Life and Activity

M.J. Mossakowski
Medical Research Centre, Polish Academy of Sciences, Warsaw, Poland

Over a year and a half has elapsed since the death of professor Stanisław Kozłowski, and still this fact seems unbelievable and certainly unacceptable. He was a man whose presence was so necessary and natural that many of us continue to think that at any moment he may come in, speak to us, telephone. . . . We expect every day to meet him, share with him our problems and joys, listen to his advice and remarks. . . . This impossibility of accepting his absence and our desire to be with him are the best evidence for who he was and what he meant to us.

Stanisław Kozłowski was born in March 1927 in Białystok and spent there the first 18 years of his life, the period of most sensitive intellectual and emotional receptivity, of development of future attitudes and ways of perceiving things, matters, and people. The climate of this rather small town situated at a specific ethnic and cultural boundary and his personal experiences during World War II and in the early postwar period deepened his perspectives, strengthened his commitments, taught him the hierarchy of values and molded his tolerance—the features so characteristic of his personality. This climate strengthened in him a feeling of group solidarity; a need for strong family, national, and cultural ties. This later found expression in his unusually deep rooting in the milieu where he worked and developed in him a strong sense of responsibility for his group as a whole and for each of its members. Participation in his youth in the patriotic activity of his province, Podlasie, strengthened him, gave him fortitude, a ready decision, and a striving for consistent realization of the goals set before him. Another factor in those years had a dominant effect on his personality—his mother, under whose influence he remained even in his mature life. I have grounds to suppose that here was the source of his attitudes toward other people, his warmth, kindness, indulgence, and benevolence.

With this background and experience Stanisław Kozłowski at the age of 18 started his studies in 1945 at the Medical Faculty of Warsaw University and graduated in 1952 with the diploma of physician. During his studies he actively participated in the intensive life of the Warsaw students' milieu, enjoying with them the newly restored possibility of studying. He shared their joys and troubles, the postwar poverty, learning the fundamental truth of those times that nothing is impossible. Crowded and unheated lecture rooms, half-ruined laboratories without necessary equipment, and the lack of manuals and lecture notes were no obstacles to intensive absorption of knowledge, when associated with true interest and motivation. Neither was the restricted space of cheap small rooms, which became even more crowded in time with the appearance of new family members, frugal meals in students' canteens, and daily privations shared by most students. The enthusiasm of Stanisław Kozłowski for learning was not even affected by the dark clouds threatening the country and university life at a time when he was midway through his studies.

In his second university year he met with what was to become the greatest fascination of his life—human physiology, to which he devoted his future—and the man who oriented his first goals and shaped the scientific career of the future professor. This man was Professor Włodzimierz Missiuro, Head of the Department of Work Physiology at the Medical School in Warsaw. Stanisław often claimed that all his intellectual and scientific life was a heritage from his teacher. Stanisław Kozłowski became bound to the department of Professor Missiuro first as a student, then as holder of a scholarship awarded by the Ministry of Health, and later as a regular staff member. He followed all the steps of a scientific career, from junior assistant to professor to head of this department.

During the years after graduation Stanisław Kozłowski finally established his scientific interests, mastering the modern continuously extending research methods and winning the rank of researcher. He supplemented his postgraduate studies by working in the Department of Internal Medicine of the Warsaw School of Medicine. This experience formally resulted in specialization in clinical physiology and strengthened the relationship between his research interests and the requirements of clinical medicine. The medical and scientific training received at his parent institutions was deepened and extended by research visits to the Department of Applied Physiology and the Clinic of Endocrinology and Metabolism of the Karolinska Institutet in Stockholm and in the Department of Physiology of the Krogh University in Copenhagen.

The contacts established with these research centers as well as with a number of other leading scientific centers in Western Europe and in the USSR evolved with time into long lasting partnerships and collaboration. The preliminary period of Stanisław Kozłowski's professional career was completed by his "habilitation" in 1966, preceded six years earlier by his doctorate obtained at the Faculty of Medicine of the School of Medicine in Warsaw. In 1968 after his teacher prof. Missiuro's death he became the Head of the Department of Exercise Physiology at the Warsaw School of Medicine, and a year later he additionally inherited the Department of Work Physiology at the Medical Research Centre of the Polish Academy of Sciences, renamed at his initiative to the Department of Applied Physiology.

Both these Departments for more than 10 years became his research battlefield, the object of his ambitions, worries, and solicitude as well as a source of his joy and pride. They became almost his home. He created a uniformly consistent group inspired by his research concepts and his vision of scientific life. Besides scientific inspiration and his attitude toward work he introduced into this group a climate of friendliness, cheerfulness, and benevolence. Having inherited rather modestly equipped traditional laboratories, he tried to modernize them. Apart from physiological techniques, he extended endocrinological and biochemical methods. Isotope and electronic laboratories were organized and a cardiological dispensary arose. Professor Kozłowski's department soon became a country-wide leading research center in Applied Physiology, well recognized by the European physiological group.

The basic subjects of prof. Stanisław Kozłowski's research comprised three main topics of Applied Physiology. The first concerned the basic mechanisms of physiological adaptation to physical effort and environmental conditions, especially the neurohormonal mechanisms of metabolic control during muscular work and its significance in developing a capability for work. The second concerned basic mechanisms of regulation of the water–electrolyte balance and thermoregulation in the organism. The third, particularly intensive in the last years of his activity, dealt with the mechanisms of exercise tolerance by people with chronic diseases of the circulatory system and metabolism and with physiological effects of cardiological rehabilitation. The results of all this work and research are presented in almost 200 original scientific papers and a dozen or so monographic publications containing a number of observations with an unshakeable value of scientific discoveries.

Professor Kozłowski knew how to teach and loved teaching. He did it with enthusiasm, finding in it personal satisfaction and pleasure. The schoolmaster's routine dryness and distance were alien to him. He was a demanding yet indulgent teacher. He was equally exacting both in respect to himself and to his students, but his indulgence and patience were reserved solely for the latter.

He was a scientist enjoying a general respect and admiration, distinguished by numerous prizes and awards and . . . a man overburdened with work. Nine years ago the first alarming warning came, but it did not change anything in prof. Kozłowski's life, which continued to be as before, active, full of successes and everyday difficulties and above all full of work. It was a mode of life he had chosen consciously and he was not ready to give up any of its attributes. It was such a rich life that it might have been sufficient for more than one man. It comprised the creative activity of a scientist, teacher, and research organizer as well as broad unprofessional interests—poetry, music, reading, and a never quenched curiosity of everything that nature and humankind created. There was a place in his life for family and friends, for creation and reflection. He knew the taste of such a life and also its price. He led the life he had chosen till the end. Only a very few succeed in doing this.

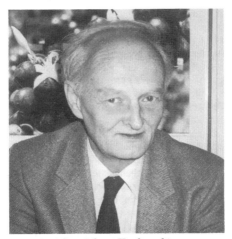

Stanisław Kozłowski

The Present State of Sports Medicine

E. Jokl

University of Kentucky, Lexington, Kentucky, United States

To understand why sport has become one of the major leisure activities of mankind, one must realize that the concepts of leisure and sport have only recently assumed their present meaning. The idea that time for leisure would be available to the common man sounded revolutionary not so long ago, when the worker, unless he was working, rested in order to recuperate and gather new strength for work. The boys and girls who slaved in coal mines and textile mills around the middle of the nineteenth century had neither the time nor the strength to play. And their as well as their elders' situation was incomparably worse than that which had prevailed during the preceding millennium in the relatively stable rural village environment predominant throughout Western Europe.

That medicine would ever become a science was beyond imagination until not so long ago, and the conquest of hunger and malnutrition is also a recent development. The role of vitamins as essential elements of a good diet was unknown until the beginning of this century. However, the greatest single contribution of medical research to society has been the increased control of infectious diseases. In 1900 infectious diseases were responsible for most deaths in the United States. Throughout the preceding centuries no family was spared the sorrow of children dying from 'fevers.' The chief causes of death in the United States today are no longer infectious diseases but cardiovascular diseases, malignant tumors, accidents, and crime. The average length of life has increased from 48 years in 1898 to 70 years today. Whooping cough, diphtheria, smallpox, and poliomyelitis were brought under control only after World War II.

It is against the background of such changes that the favorable status of children today must be assessed. Today's boys and girls are taller and stronger than their parents and grandparents. An average-sized high school boy aged 17 would not fit into the armor of Elizabethan knights in the Tower of London. There has been a steady acceleration of growth and maturation over the centuries, with a noticeable spurt during the past decades. One manifestation of this spurt is the appearance of children and adolescents in sports such as swimming, gymnastics, ice skating, and other athletic disciplines. Children nowadays run the 26-mile marathon, climb the highest mountains, and participate in long-distance ski races. Sixteen-year-old Ulrike Meyfarth won the high jump at the Munich Olympic Games in 1972. At the 1976 Olympic Games in Montreal, 15-year-old Nadja Comaneci dominated the gymnastic competition, while 16-year-old Cornelia Ender won four gold medals in the swimming events.

Concurrent with the acceleration of growth is a deceleration of aging, a phenomenon that is the physiological basis for the participation of large numbers of older men and women in a great variety of sporting events. The Swiss statistician Carl Schneiter reported that the running times of men 50 to 60 years old in the ski marathon in St. Moritz were significantly better in 1985 than in 1975, showing that the deceleration of aging as a determinant of endurance continues.

The athletic status of women reflects the far reaching changes that have taken place in the Western world during this century. During the past 50 years, millions of girls have become engaged in sports, gymnastics, and games; have competed in swimming, track and field events, and horseback riding; have climbed many of the highest mountains and have swum through a thousand rivers and lakes. They have derived therefrom some of the most valuable experiences of their lives.

That the present generation of women grows stronger; that their physical maturation is better balanced; that their appearance has become more attractive; that the state of health of young mothers and their children today is superior; that physically active women no longer look old at the age of 30; that many schoolgirls play on the same teams as their mothers; all this is, at least in part, the result of the interest now taken in the physical education of girls. Sports and games and athletics for women are significant elements of what is best in contemporary culture.

Although the advances of science and technology have resulted in the conquest of hunger and the control of infectious diseases, not more than a quarter of the world's total population has yet benefited from them. The medical status of most of the populations of Asia and Africa today is no better than it was in Europe during the Middle Ages. The extent to which infectious diseases affect the physical status of entire ethnic groups became evident during the past 20 years in East Africa when smallpox was eradicated through the use of vaccination. Only then did Hamitic athletes from Tanzania, Ethiopia, and Kenya appear on the international athletic scene. Conspicuous successes at the 1972 Olympic Games established their countries as major track and field powers. Their status will continue to improve as additional public health measures become effective. A worldwide upgrading of all sports performances is bound to take place when the results of preventive and curative measures that are currently introduced by the World Health Organization throughout the Third World become noticeable. During the next two decades public health measures are likely to reduce the incidence of all diseases everywhere.

Technological innovations will also play an important role in the athletic performance explosion of our century. The introduction of Tartan tracks, newly designed javelins and discuses, fiberglass poles, and foam rubber mats have noticeably altered the track and field scene. Temperature control of swimming pools, improved filtration systems, and establishment of smooth water surfaces through vertical lane markers have improved swimming records. The availability of large indoor facilities, such as the air-conditioned Astrodome in Houston and the Louisiana Superdome in New Orleans, has provided the opportunity for creating optimal room temperatures and other advantageous environmental conditions for individual athletic events throughout the year. And last but not least, the fact that numbers of participants in all sports are continually increasing throughout the world renders probable the appearance from time to time of "athletic geniuses" and thus the establishment of extraordinary records.

Once the limits of physical performance growth are reached, a chief objective of athletics will be to explore the esthetic possibilities inherent in sport, possibilities derived from the inexhaustible choice of designs of expression and communication of human movement. Through the unprecedented differentiation of the motor system, which sport in all its manifestations is capable of accomplishing, sport is destined to reveal its powers of experience and communication.

How Useful Is Knowledge of Work Physiology in the Modern World?

H. Monod

Centre National de la Recherche Scientifique, Paris, France

Work physiology, exercise physiology, the physiology of people at work, and industrial physiology are terms used by physiologists in their descriptions of people involved in sporting or professional activities. This approach differs markedly from that generally employed in trials conducted by physicians, where pathology is evaluated in light of the physiology of subjects at rest in bed. What are the human capacities for adaptation to exercise, what mechanisms and limits are involved, what are the immediate or longer term effects of increased muscular activity, and how can physical aptitude be assessed and increased?

The Aims of Work Physiology

There are at least three: (a) to improve understanding, (b) to teach or exchange knowledge in work physiology, and (c) to develop methods and tools for research and its applications. The first aim of work physiology is to improve our understanding of various aspects of people in their occupational environment. Data are available regarding respiratory, cardiovascular, and energetic adaptations. The relationships between the main biological parameters and exercise power are well established. In contrast, some physiological data are incomplete, such as the relationship between the type of foodstuff and sporting performance and the endocrine regulation of energy metabolism.

Numerous countries have laboratories for the investigation of work physiology, muscular exercise, sport exercise, fatigue, or human performance. The importance of such laboratories has, on occasion, been called into question due to reductionist tendencies in modern biology (i.e., a strong preference for molecular biology). It is perhaps in the field of work physiology that the need for an integrated approach is most apparent.

The second aim of work physiology is to facilitate the exchange of data required for the training of specialists in industrial biology, ergonomics, rehabilitation, physical education, and kinesiology. Numerous universities offer courses in specific subjects that may not always be officially recognized. Furthermore, scientific meetings provide an excellent outlet for the exchange of information, as do specialized journals.

Finally, work physiology aims to address two present-day problems: (a) In terms of sport and leisure—how can the sportsperson's activity be organized; how can events be won and how can champions be produced? and (b) In terms of the consumer society—how can hazard-free goods fulfilling human requirements be produced without involving excessive fatigue for the worker? These two questions overlap in terms of the determination of the mental and physical aptitude of sportsmen and women or workers for a given activity.

The Development of Work Physiology

Work physiology has progressed markedly since the beginning of this century due to technical advances in electronics and computing and the development of new noninvasive exploratory methods (Kayser, 1947). This progress may create the illusion that physiological studies of men and women involved in various activities are easy and can be carried out by a technician with an average training. However, this overlooks the important role played by physiological reasoning, which is essential for the organization and completion of research projects and the discussion of results.

Physiological Exploration

Physiological exploration employs the same methods for all subjects from marathon runners to lumberjacks. However, the marathon runner is motivated by the need to run as fast as possible for 2-1/2 hours. Such exercise calls for a high mobilization of aerobic power, whereas the lumberjack must perform professional tasks every day for months or years, pacing daily aerobic output at a reasonable percentage of his or her aerobic capacity. Physiological exploration of human activity has focussed in particular on the determination of energy consumption and heart rate.

The consideration of people at work as machines involved in energy exchanges has long been a cornerstone of work physiology, as shown by the studies of certain physiologists, who are rightly considered in France as the forerunners of present-day work physiologists (Amar, 1914; Bert, 1867-1868; Marey, 1873). The development of devices for the measurement of energy consumption has been stimulated by the need for evaluation of the physical work involved in industrial production and in the mandatory physical training of the armed forces, and increasing standards in sports competitions. They include the Douglas bag, the portable devices of Kofranyi-Michaelis, and of Muller, and the IMP (the integrating motor pneumotechygraph) device.

Because of technical difficulties in the measurement of oxygen consumption in exercising subjects, work physiologists have gradually turned their attention to the simpler measurement of heart rate (see Merklen, 1926). Energy consumption and heart rate are related by a simple mathematical expression, with uncertainty due to variability in the stroke volume and reduction in venous oxygen to below saturation levels.

The measurement of heart rate by palpation of the radial pulse, which leads to calculation of the cardiac cost of the work done (cardiac equivalent of net oxygen consumption), has advanced greatly following the studies of Brouha (1963) in heavy industry. Electrocardiography and photoplethysmography have improved conditions for observation of cardiac activity, but the mobility of the tested subject remained insufficient (see Monod, 1967).

Physiological Reasoning

A good understanding of work physiology is necessary in order to avoid certain errors of interpretations and to temper the enthusiasm engendered by easily acquired recordings. The evaluation of maximal oxygen consumption from the Åstrand (1952) nomogram is both common and highly useful. It should be remembered, however, that there is much space between the measurement and the assessment of physiological parameters. For instance, the individual or population studied differs from the population for which the nomogram was drawn up (degree of training, and so on). Similarly, the correction of values as a function of age uses a theoretical, not real, maximal heart rate value.

Evaluation of energy consumption during a sport or professional activity involves the plotting of heart rates, determined during exercise, on a standard individual straight line previously drawn up on the basis of laboratory values for oxygen consumption–heart rate determined for increasing power. The approach is interesting but can provide only relative information since the test conditions differ in the laboratory and in the field. The differences involve the active muscle groups, posture, climatic conditions, and the time of day.

Would it be easier to reason only on the basis of heart rate rather than on presumed values of energy consumption? It should be recalled that the so-called resting heart rate is unprecise and even if accurate it is inadequate to consider heart rate values alone. During a normal male lifespan of 77 years, the heart beats approximately 2.7×10^9 times for a sedentary subject and 2.8×10^9 times for a worker involved in heavy labor, that is, an increase of 4% for the latter. This difference should not be viewed as paltry, even though this overlooks the high blood pressure at which the heart is forced to work. As a general rule, excessive importance should not be attached to a single physiological criterion.

One question that arises concerns the meaning that can be attached to a physical aptitude test. These tests can assume various forms: determination of maximal exercise power when the subject works at full capacity; study of physiological reactions during calibrated exercise (the best subjects are those with the most moderate physiological reactions). A given test can be used for various purposes when comparing a given individual under two different sets of conditions: before and after some weeks of training and before and after some hours of sporting or professional activity. In the latter case the aptitude test becomes a fatigue test. Finally, it should be noted that the test reflects the real work capacity of an individual from only one angle: The coach or physician should accord it only a relative value. As for laboratory research scientists who seek to understand the underlying causative mechanisms, they should bear in mind that not all their assumptions are equally easy to verify.

Conclusions

The above considerations have shown that work physiology is a genuine and vital part of physiology, notably of applied physiology. In parallel with physiologists who are oriented toward functional studies of pathological subjects, work and sport physiologists devote their attention to the study of healthy subjects. Fortunately, normal healthy subjects are in the great majority in today's world.

References

Amar, J. (1914). *Le moteur humain*. Dunod et Pinat, Paris.
Åstrand, P.O. (1952). *Experimental studies of physical working capacity in relation to sex and age*. Munksgaard, Copenhagen.
Bert, P. (1867-1868). *La machine humaine*. Hachette, Paris.
Brouha, L. (1963). *Physiologie et industrie*. Gauthier-Villars, Paris.
Kayser, C. (1947). *Physiologie du travail et du sport*. Herman, Paris.
Marey, J.E. (1873). *La machine animale*. Baillière, Paris.
Merklen, L. (1926). *Le rythme du coeur au cours de l'activité musculaire et notamment des exercise sportifs*. Camille André, Nancy.
Monod, H. (1967). *La validité des mesures de fréquence cardiaque en ergonomie*. Ergonomics, London.

Part I
Cardiovascular Adjustments and Adaptation to Physical Exercise

The Frontiers Between Physiology and Pathology in the Athlete's Heart: To What Limits Can It Enlarge and Beat Slowly?

R. Rost

Institute for Sports Medicine, University of Dortmund, F.R.G.

The athlete's heart (AH) is certainly one of the oldest and most stimulating subjects for research in sports medicine. The first credit for having described it belongs to Henschen in the late 19th century. However, in the long history of sportsmedical research, there has never been as much controversy on any subject than on the interpretation of AH as a physiological phenomenon. Its assessment was always a scientific tug-of-war between those who viewed it as a physiologically adapted, extremely effective and healthy heart, and those who regarded it as a sick heart or, at least, a heart on the borderline of pathology.

The frequent interpretation of the AH as a sick organ is readily understandable regarding its outstanding size and its functional properties, training bradycardia of as low as 20 beats/min being the most impressive among them. The physiologist observes an enlargement as an indication of incipient failure. For him, an enlarging heart is always a negative sign. The assumption that "a large heart is a sick heart," when applied to the AH, is based on the lack of recognition that in physiological experiments the adaptation factor of cardiac enlargement is missing. The clinician frequently fails to recognize the fact that in the athlete the enlargement of the heart also denotes an improvement of its performance, as it was already underlined by Henschen (1899).

Henschen (1899) observed in cross-country skiers that "big hearts win the races" and, therefore, he concluded that "an enlarged heart is a good thing, if it can perform more work over an extended period of time." Even if this conclusion seems to be self-evident, a controversial discussion of the AH can be seen through its almost century-long history after Henschen. Only a few examples of the misgivings on the AH should be mentioned:

Shortly after Henschen, Moritz (1902) tried to equate AH with his ideas of tonogenic and myogenic dilatation. Later authors considered it to be the result of preexistent weakness and a development on the basis of Starling's law, for example, overexertion (Deutsch & Kauf, 1924; Kaufmann, 1933; Lysholm et al., 1934). The most surprising interpretation can be found in the standard American cardiology textbook by Friedberg which, even in the 1972 edition, made the statement that the AH has to be interpreted as a result of overexertion in a rheumatic, syphilitic, or congenitally damaged heart. Keren and Schoenfeld (1981) concluded that sudden death may be more frequent as a result of those changes that can be covered by the term "athlete's heart syndrome."

The main well-known symptoms of this "syndrome" are cardiac hypertrophy and bradycardia. The questions of how far these changes can be considered as physiological and whether the borderline of the physiological area may be surpassed by training results will be discussed subsequently. Concerning hypertrophy it should be stressed that this problem has been widely discussed and satisfactorily concluded in the German literature from 1930 to 1960. Morphological studies in athletes who died suddenly by noncardiac reasons became the basis of this discussion. We must still depend on the data of Kirch, who was the first and up to now the only one who performed such investigations. Kirch published autopsy findings of 35 athletes in 1935 and 1936. According to him an overproportional hypertrophy of the heart can be caused by physical exercise.

This was not accepted by other pathologists, such as Aschoff (1928), who recognized cardiac enlargement as a consequence of general physical conditioning, and not as a particular adaptational mechanism. Kirch found no evidence of cardiac damage that could be attributed to physical training; however, the weight of the hearts examined by him never exceeded 500 g, a limit that was called a "critical heart weight" by Linzbach (1958). Another important point from the findings of Kirch is the fact that the hypertrophy does not always need to be symmetrical and that preferential enlargement of the right or left heart could be observed. In most cases, though, the right ventricular hypertrophy predominates, in accordance with the high incidence of an incomplete right bundle-branch block in the athlete's ECG. Kirch was unable to assign these differences in hypertrophy to any specific athletic activity.

Even if the form of hypertrophy might not depend on the type of sport, it certainly applies for the degree of enlargement. This was demonstrated by radiological investigations that replaced the morphological assessment of the AH, which fortunately cannot be performed in athletes as a routine method. Radiological measurement of cardiac volume was introduced by Scandinavian authors Rohrer (1916), Kahlstorf (1933), and Kjellberg et al. (1949) (Figure 1). Reindell et al. (1960) combined this technique with the functional evaluation of cardiac performance measured as maximum oxygen uptake. Such investigations demonstrated an average cardiac volume in male subjects of 11 ml/kg body weight. Cardiac enlargement depends on the endurance type of training (Figure 2). The largest hearts are found in endurance athletes such as runners and cyclists, and no influence is to be seen in sprinters, weightlifters, or gymnasts. Cardiac enlargement correlates closely with the maximum oxygen uptake, thus substantiating the old statement from Henschen of the big heart winning the race.

Summarizing the old literature we can answer the question, Up to what limit can the AH enlarge? as follows: physiological hypertrophy is only found in endurance athletes; it always stops at a critical heart weight of 500 g; and it never changes to a pathological process.

These old answers have to be challenged in 1987 from two points of view: (a) Since the investigations of Kirch, training intensity has risen to an extreme degree (the athletes examined by him were only moderately trained and some of them might be considered as being only leisure-time athletes), and (b) new methods, particularly echocardiography, have brought about new insights.

The questions to be asked are: (a) Is there really a "critical heart weight," and if so, is this limit still the same as in the 1930s or do we have to accept higher values regarding the extreme cardiac load in modern athletes? (b) If there is a critical heart weight, does this mean an absolute value, or would it be preferable to accept an individual value regarding different body size and genetical determination of the athletes? (c) Critical heart weight implies a danger if this limit were to be exceeded. Does this concept have to be accepted, and where is the risk to be looked for? (d) Echocardiography has produced new findings about training effects in the heart of the "power" athletes. Morganroth et al. (1975) was the first to describe a "pure concentric hypertrophy" in the hearts of weight-lifters. Do we have to assume a specific form of physiological hypertrophy for different types of athletics? and (e) Echocardiography has also brought about some new aspects of pathological forms of hypertrophy, such as hypertrophic cardiomyopathy (HCM). Maron et al. (1980) found HCM to be a major reason for sudden death in athletes. May it be possible that physiological hypertrophy favors the development of pathological forms, at least in the case of a congenital disposition?

If we consider the concept of a critical heart weight as the assumption that physiological hypertrophy must have its reasonable limits, then this model makes sense. In spite of the

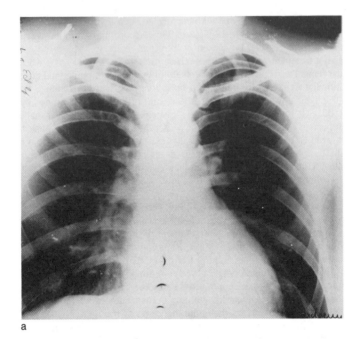

a

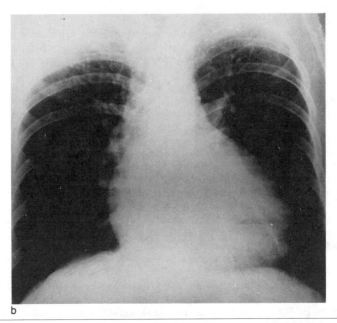

b

Figure 1. (a) X-ray presentation of an AH in the normal standing position. (b) X-ray presentation of an AH in supine position to measure cardiac volume. In this case the heart of a professional cycling champion had a cardiac volume of 1500 ml.

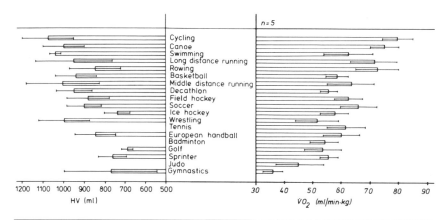

Figure 2. Relation of cardiac volume (left side) and relative maximum oxygen uptake (right side) in top-ranking athletes.

tremendous increase in training intensity, we do not find larger hearts in athletes than Reindell et al. did in the 1950s using the same radiological techniques. The largest AH were found to be 1700 ml in a water polo player (Medved & Friedrich, 1964) and in a professional cyclist (Hollmann, 1965). Related to body weight, the highest value (20.8 ml/kg) was found by Reindell in a long-distance runner. Even if world records remarkably increased within the last two decades, the AH did not. Physiological hypertrophy ends at a reasonable limit, and further increase of performance has to be based on metabolic, not on hemodynamic, adaptations.

Another aspect of intensified training in top athletics is the shift of training and competition to childhood. In endurance sports this particularly concerns swimming. As the major cause of the maintenance of a upper limit in physiological hypertrophy, generally the inability of cardiac muscle to become hyperplastic after birth is accentuated. Therefore, regarding the greater plasticity of the younger heart, the early start of competitive training today may lead to AH larger than those seen to date. To substantiate this hypothesis we followed a group of children beginning high-intensity training before puberty over more than one decade, applying echocardiography and radiological investigations. Even in those children we could not find larger hearts than were found before in swimmers. In conclusion: Even in a very early onset of top training the limits of physiological hypertrophy are maintained.

This experience with top athletes supports the opinion of Linzbach (1958) and others that physiological hypertrophy takes place in a restricted form only. Another problem is the dogmatical maintenance of a upper limit of 500 g. The largest heart in the athletes described by Kirch belonged to a professional boxer, its weight being 530 g. According to our experience these athletes never exceeded a cardiac volume of 1200 ml. It seems unlikely that the hearts of 1700 ml observed by Hollmann (1965) or Medved and Friedrich (1964) were not heavier than that. On the other hand, maximum cardiac enlargements should also depend on individual characteristics. It seems to be self-evident to accept a higher maximum in larger athletes; otherwise, logically, the trainability would be larger in smaller athletes. Measuring the left ventricular muscle mass (LVM) by two-dimensional echocardiography, Dickhuth et al. (1985) assumed a harmonious hypertrophy (LVM being 47% of the total heart weight). Regarding these conditions, they used a "relative maximum critical heart weight" of 7.5 g/kg body weight. Even if the absolute values in large athletes may be too high (a 100-kg rower could have a heart weight up to 750 g), this concept seems to be sensible. Perhaps it would be better to refer the relative maximum heart weight to body surface.

Another individual factor that might define the endpoint of maximum physiological hypertrophy is heredity. A large heart is considered to be a major attribute of an "endurance-talent;" however, unfortunately, nobody assesses these athletes before the start of training. Therefore, this problem, which is of extreme importance for the selection of "talents," remains open for discussion.

What makes critical heart weight critical? It is frequently argued that the inability of hyperplasia may limit physiological hypertrophy since hypertrophy leads to an increase in the diffusion pathway for oxygen to the center of the myocardial fiber. However, the question of myocardial hyperplasia is not yet answered conclusively. Linzbach (1958) emphasized the fact that the number of cardiac muscle fibers remains constant in physiological hypertrophy, but he did not exclude hyperplasia. He assumed additional factors such as coronary insufficiency creating "structural dilation" after exceeding critical heart weight, a condition absent in healthy athletes. Under similar prerequisites, young people with chronic volume overload, such as aortic insufficiency, may exceed critical heart weight without any signs of cardiac failure. By these reasons the upper limit observed in athletes is not really critical, and therefore the term critical heart weight should be replaced by a term such as maximum physiological hypertrophy.

As already mentioned, echocardiographic investigations stimulated discussion on particular forms of physiological hypertrophy even in power athletes. Morganroth et al. (1975) described a concentric hypertrophy in these athletes in contrast to a "pure dilation" in endurance athletes, a concept that seems to be reasonable regarding the predominant volume work during dynamic exercise in contrast to the increased pressure work during the static effort. Yet, on pure theoretical grounds the simple distinction cannot be correct. According to Laplace's law, each enlargement of ventricular diameter under physiological conditions has to be accompanied by a thickening of myocardial wall. Therefore, cardiac enlargement found in endurance athletes does not correspond to a pure dilation but to the eccentric hypertrophy, as it was already described in other terms by Henschen (1899), and then convincingly demonstrated by echocardiography. We could not confirm the concentric hypertrophy in power athletes (Figures 3 & 4). Of course, there are some examples of such type of hypertrophy in power athletes, but this can also be found for unknown reasons in endurance athletes. A recent two-dimensional study gave the same result (Dickhuth et al., 1985).

The occasional observation of concentric hypertrophy raises the question whether physiological hypertrophy may lead to pathological forms of hypertrophy. Actually, sometimes it may be rather difficult to distinguish such forms of physiological hypertrophy from the beginning of HCM, particularly if they appear simultaneously with repolarization abnormalities, which are seen in the athlete's ECG as well. On the other hand, there is no reason to assume such a possibility of HCM stimulation by training since, otherwise, there should be a higher incidence of this disease in trained people.

In summary, even today, in regards to the extreme intensity of modern top athletics we have to confirm the old opinion that physiological hypertrophy always remains within restricted borderlines. This hypertrophy takes place in a uniform way as eccentric hypertrophy, and there is no sufficient proof to accept concentric hypertrophy in certain types of sports. In contrast to some older hypotheses, maximum physiological hypertrophy should not be considered in terms of a really critical limit, since it seems to be an individual rather than an absolute variable.

The question, to what limits AH can beat slowly, is easily answered by the number 21, the lowest heart rate in an athlete so far published in the literature. Zeppilli and Venerando (1981) found this value by Holter monitoring; the lowest heart rate we recorded was 25.

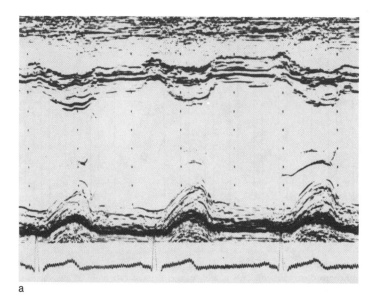

a

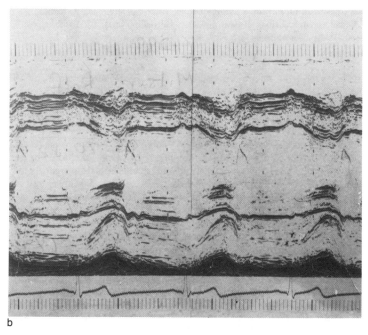

b

Figure 3. Examples of M-mode presentation of athlete's hearts. (a) Example of an endurance athlete, a world champion in professional cycling, demonstrating an extreme left ventricular diameter of 70 mm and only a modest hypertrophy of left ventricular wall. (b) "Typical" concentric hypertrophy in a power athlete, a world champion weight lifter.

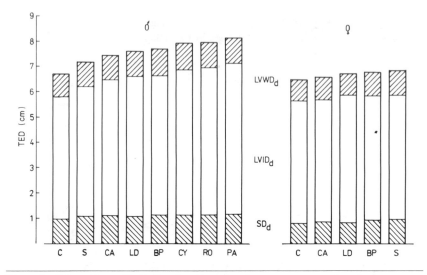

Figure 4. Echocardiographic findings in athletes that demonstrate more or less the same type of hypertrophy in all subsamples. Abbreviations: TED (total end-diastolic diameter), LVWD$_d$ (left ventricular back-wall diameter), LVID (left ventricular internal diameter), SD$_d$ (septal thickness), all measured during diastole. Athletic subsamples: C (control), S (swimmers), CA (canoeists), LD (long distance runners), BP (ballplayers), CY (cyclists), RO (rowers), PA (power athletes).

Generally, however, heart rate in athletes is not as low. By Holter monitoring of 50 endurance athletes, we have found the lowest heart rate in the majority of them between 40-50, only in 12 between 30-40, and in none under 30. It is surprising that such very low heart rates are generally based on a regular sinus rhythm. Israel (1975) has pointed out that escape rhythm is relatively rare. The degree of bradycardia is, in contrast to cardiac enlargement, a rather poor measure of the level of training. Very low rates can be also found occasionally in nontrained persons who have a high vagal tone. According to Roskamm et al. (1966), among nine German national teams, the gymnasts had surprisingly the lowest heart rates, even though these athletes have a comparatively low cardiovascular capacity.

Although training bradycardia is a very striking phenomenon, it has not been adequately elucidated to date. Frequently it is interpreted as a result of cardiac enlargement, for example, as a consequence of a high stroke volume. However, this assessment does not fit the poor correlation between training bradycardia and cardiovascular performance. To escape this problem an increased vagal tone is made responsible for bradycardia. However, if this were true, a vagal tone lowering heart rate to 30 beats/min should also have been found in noncardiac areas.

Animal experiments are helpful for understanding of bradycardia. Tipton (1965) found a decrease in heart rate in the denervated hearts of rats. According to his results heart rate is diminished, not through an increase in the vagal tone, but by an increased sensitivity of the heart to vagal stimulation. The atrial muscle of the trained rat contains an increased concentration of nonneural acetylcholine.

From the clinical point of view, the most important question is the borderline of heart rate that can be tolerated by AH without clinical symptoms. In the endurance-trained athlete an increased stroke volume can compensate, without any difficulty, for the decreased heart rate. It is the common experience of all sports medicine centers that even extreme bradycardia in athletes is well tolerated. This statement is in clear contrast to a clinical study published by Ector et al. (1984). They observed 16 athletes suffering from syncope, 3 of them even suffered a cardiac arrest, and in 7, pacemakers were implanted. However, since this experience is contradictory to all sport–cardiological experiences (we do not know any athletes needing a pacemaker), probably this study describes not athletes having trouble with training bradycardia, but patients with arrhythmias who were exercising. Sufficient information about training intensity was not given in that study. On the other hand, this observation underlines the fact that training results may lead to problems when there is subclinical damage. It seems to be probable that in the case of slight sinus or AV defects, additional vagotonic effects may produce clinical symptoms. Particularly, some of the increasing numbers of elderly people performing endurance training today may suffer from a latent sick sinus syndrome or AV block and really run into problems or even need a pacemaker. Summing up, training bradycardia is a physiological phenomenon very well tolerated by the AH, but sometimes it may accentuate subclinical symptoms.

References

Aschoff, L. (1928). Die anatomischen Grundlagen von der Herzvergrösserung und der muskulären Herzschwäche. Verh. 4, S. 62. Dtsch. Sportärztetagung Berlin 1927. Fischer, Jena.

Deutsch, F., & Kauf, E. (1924). Herz und Sport. Wien-Bern.

Dickhuth, H., Jakob, E., Wink, K., Bonzel, T., Keul, J., & Just, H. (1985). Lässt sich aus der maximalen Herzhypertrophie ein absolutes kritisches Herzgewicht ableiten? In J. Franz, H. Mellerowicz, & W. Noack (Hrsg.), Training und Sport zur Prävention und Rehabilitation in der technischen Umwelt. Springer, Berlin, Heidelberg, New York, Tokyo, 722.

Ector, H., Bourgois, J., Verlinden, M., Hermans, L., Van Den Eyne, E., Fagard, R., & De Geest, H. (1984). Bradycardia, ventricular pauses, syncope, and sports. Lancet II, 591.

Friedberg, C. (1972). Erkrankungen des Herzens. 2. Aufl., Thieme, Stuttgart.

Henschen, S. (1899). Skilanglauf und Skiwettlauf. Eine medizinische Sportstudie. Mitt. med. Klin., Upsala, Jena.

Hollmann, W. (1965). Körperliches Training als Prävention von Herz-Kreislauf-Krankheiten. Hippokrates Verlag, Stuttgart.

Israel, S. (1975). Die Herzfunktion bei trainingsbedingten extremen Bradykardien von 29-34 min⁻¹. Med. u. Sport, 15, 197.

Kahlstorf, A. (1933). Uber Korrelationen der linearen Herzmasse und des Herzvolumens. Klin. Wschr., 12, 262.

Kaufmann, W. (1933). Die Beeinflussung der Herzgrösse durch Arbeit und Sport. Med. Welt., 7, 1347.

Keren, G., & Schoenfeld, Y. (1981). Sudden death and physical exertion. J. Sports Med., 21, 90.

Kirch, E. (1935). Anatomische Grundlagen des Sportherzens. Verh. Dtsch. Ges. Inn. Med., 47, 73.

Kirch, E. (1936). Herzkräftigung und echte Herzhypertrophie durch Sport. Z. Kreislauff, 28, 893.

Kjellberg, S., Ruhde, U., & Sjøstrand, T. (1949). The relation of the cardiac volume to the weight and surface area of the body, the blood volume and the physical capacity for work. Acta Radiol., 31, 115.

Linzbach, A. (1958). Struktur und Funktion des gesunden und kranken Herzens. In Die Funktionsdiagnostik des Herzens, S. 94, H. Klepzig (Hrsg.). Springer Verlag, Berlin, Göttingen, Heidelberg.

Lysholm, E., Nylin, G., & Quarna, K. (1934). The relation between heart volume and stroke volume under physiological and pathological conditions. Acta Radiol., 15, 237.

Maron, B., Roberts, W., McAllister, H., Rosing, D., & Epstein, S. (1980). Sudden death in young athletes. *Circulation*, **62**, 218.

Medved, R., & Friedrich, V. (1964). The largest athletic heart recorded in the literature. *Lijecnicki Vjesnik* (medical journal), **86**, 843.

Morganroth, J., Maron, B., Henry, W., & Epstein, S. (1975). Comparative left ventricular dimensions in trained athletes. *Ann. Int. Med.*, **82**, 521.

Moritz, F. (1902). Über orthodiagraphische Untersuchungen am Herzen. *Med. Wschr.*, **49**(1), 1.

Reindell, H., Klepzig, H., Steim, H., Musshoff, K., Roskamm, H., & Schildge, E. (1960). *Herz-Kreislaufkrankheiten und Sport*. Barth, München.

Rohrer, F. (1916). Volumenbestimmungen an Körperöhlen und Organen auf orthodiagraphischem Wege. *Fortschr. Röntgenstr.*, **24**, 285.

Roskamm, H., Reindell, H., & Müller, M. (1966). Herzgrösse und ergometrisch getestete Ausdauerleistungsfähigkeit bei Hochleistungssportlern aus 9 deutschen Nationalmannschaften. *Z. Kreislauff*, **55**, 2.

Rost, R. (1987). *Athletics and the heart*. Year Book Medical Publishers, Chicago, London.

Tipton, C. (1965). Training and bradycardia in rats. *Am. J. Physiol.*, **208**, 480.

Zeppilli, P., & Venerando, A. (1981). Sudden death and physical exertion. *J. Sports Med.*, **21**, 299.

The Influence of Exercise Training on Muscle Blood Flow

R.L. Terjung, R.M. McAllister, and B. Mackie-Engbretson

State University of New York, Health Science Center, Syracuse, New York

Endurance type exercise training induces significant increases in exercise performance, evident by an increase in maximal aerobic work capacity and an improvement in endurance performance during prolonged submaximal exercise. Associated with these training adaptations are significant cardiovascular changes which lead to altered muscle function. An increase in peak muscle blood flow as well as microvascular changes within the active muscle should serve to improve aerobic work capacity and muscle performance. This paper will consider relevant data directed at answering three questions: (a) Does training increase maximal blood flow capacity of muscle? (b) Do adaptations occur within muscle to enhance blood/tissue exchange properties? and (c) Are these adaptations important in the functional improvement in muscle performance?

Training-Induced Changes in Muscle Blood Flow Capacity

The increase in maximal oxygen consumption, typical of exercise training, has been attributed both to an increase in maximal cardiac output and to an increase in oxygen extraction from the arterial blood (cf. Clausen, 1976). The greater cardiac output leads to an increase in oxygen delivery to the periphery and, when directed to the working muscles, should lead to an increase in work capacity and maximal oxygen consumption. Thus, a greater peak blood flow to the working muscle is anticipated after training. Exceptionally high muscle blood flows should be evident in selected trained individuals who have very high aerobic capacities (Ekblom & Hermansen, 1968). Until recently, however, this expectation was without direct experimental evidence. Determination of muscle blood flow during maximal flow conditions involving whole body exercise in vivo is technically difficult and/or open to measurement limitations. For example, muscle blood flows determined with the xenon washout technique lead to significant underestimates, especially at high flow rates (Cerretelli et al., 1984). Indirect evidence, however, is available. A training-induced increased capacity for vasodilation has been obtained by indirect means such as venous occlusion plethysmography (Snell et al., 1987). Such evidence implies that physical training leads to a greater peak muscle blood flow during maximal aerobic exercise. Direct measurement of muscle blood flow has been obtained in trained rats during whole body exercise using the radiolabeled microsphere technique. However, the exercise condition employed at the time of blood flow determination was at a submaximal intensity (Armstrong & Laughlin, 1984). While differences in blood flow distribution were found between trained and sedentary animals, it is not possible to gain insight about training-induced changes in peak blood flows to muscle.

Blood Flow During Maximal Exercise In Vivo

To our knowledge, only one experimental study has employed a direct assessment of muscle blood flow during maximal exercise. Musch et al. (1987) determined blood flow using radiolabeled microspheres during maximal treadmill running in foxhounds. This study is most significant since comparisons can be made within the same animal before and after training. The training program increased maximal oxygen consumption by approximately 30% (to 149 ± 5 ml/min/kg). A similar increase in cardiac output (28%) was observed. Blood flow to the hindlimb locomotory muscles was significantly greater following training, by approximately 10%, than the peak flow measured during maximal aerobic exercise before training. Thus, exercise training resulted in an increase in peak blood flow to the working muscles during maximal whole body exercise. Interestingly, an increase in blood flow to other muscles, that may have been relatively unused during maximal running prior to training, must have also occurred. This increase in blood flow was likely due to a greater recruitment of ancillary muscles during the more strenuous exercise conditions necessary to elicit the higher maximal oxygen consumption after training. Thus, the large increase in maximal oxygen consumption was achieved by the greater cardiac output used to perfuse not only a greater muscle mass but the primary hindlimb locomotory muscles at a higher blood flow. While extensive data are not yet available, it is likely that the above conclusion is applicable in the broadest sense to most training situations where there is an increase in maximal oxygen consumption and cardiac output.

An increase in peak muscle blood flow could be due to two factors, a greater capacity of the vascular circuit or a greater dilation of the resistance vessels. Unfortunately, it is not possible from the data of Musch et al. (1987) to determine which factor leads to the training-induced increase in peak blood flow observed in the hindlimb locomotory muscles of the dogs. In order to evaluate this possible training response, it is essential to determine muscle blood flow during conditions designed to create maximal vascular dilation when central cardiovascular factors are not limiting. A limited muscle mass contracting maximally should establish an appropriate experimental system since perfusion pressure can easily be maintained and muscle contractions are a potent stimulus for vasodilation (Laughlin & Armstrong, 1985). This goal was achieved with stimulation of the gastrocnemius-plantaris-soleus muscle group of the rat in situ (Mackie & Terjung, 1983b). An increase in blood flow to an apparent peak asymptotic flow during increasingly intense stimulation conditions should identify the blood flow capacity of the muscle. Use of the rat model was also valuable in that potential training-induced alterations in blood flow capacity to the different skeletal muscle fiber type sections could be determined. In most nonprimate mammalian skeletal muscles there are fairly distinct regions composed of primarily one fiber type. Blood flows during contractions vary significantly between skeletal muscle fiber sections. Blood flows are relatively high in the high oxidative fast-twitch red and slow-twitch red fiber sections and relatively low in the fast-twitch white muscle fiber section (Laughlin & Armstrong, 1985; Mackie & Terjung, 1983a). In addition, the different skeletal muscle fiber types are recruited during exercise in a manner generally dependent on the intensity of exercise. Thus, changes in blood flow capacity induced by training in a specific fiber type region could have a significant influence on muscle performance, depending upon the intensity of exercise.

Blood Flow in Different Skeletal Muscle Fiber Type Sections After Training

Mackie and Terjung (1983b) found no significant difference in peak blood flows between sedentary and trained high oxidative fast-twitch red muscle sections even during intense stimulation conditions. These contraction conditions would have increased oxygen consumption of this muscle section by at least 30-fold (Hood et al., 1986). While a higher blood flow was apparent in the trained fast-twitch red muscle section during mild stimulation conditions, the absolute values were no greater than that observed at the most severe stimulation condition. Similarly, no training effect was found for peak blood flow in the slow-twitch red muscle. However, the peak blood flow observed in the fast-twitch white muscle section of the trained muscle was significantly greater (by approximately 45%) than the corresponding section of the sedentary muscle (Mackie & Terjung, 1983b). This response can be interpreted as an increase in blood flow capacity, due for example to an enlarged vascular circuit, since blood flow in this section was constant over a broad range of contraction conditions designed to optimize vasodilation. Additional evidence of an increased capacity of the vascular circuit in the muscles of trained animals comes from the work of Laughlin and Ripperger (1987). Training significantly increased vascular conductance of an isolated perfused hindquarter preparation maximally dilated with papaverine. Thus, it is concluded that the flow capacity of the vascular circuit of muscle can be increased by exercise training. Yet, as discussed below, this does not appear to be an essential adaptation leading to an increase in muscle blood flow after training.

Peak Muscle Conductance During Maximal Exercise in Humans

Recent work has provided convincing evidence that the peak muscle blood flow observed during maximal whole body exercise is well below the capacity of the vascular circuit of the muscle even in normal individuals. Saltin and co-workers (Anderson & Saltin, 1985; Rowell et al., 1986; Saltin, 1985) have reported exceptionally high muscle blood flows to the quadriceps muscle during strenuous single-leg knee extension exercise. The working muscle mass was kept relatively small so that essentially all of the cardiac output reserve would be available to perfuse this muscle group. The quadriceps vascular conductance could be increased even further by hypoxia as long as the cardiac reserve was not exhausted (Rowell, 1986). However, if a larger muscle mass is maximally exercising, there is a greater "competition" for the available cardiac output, and actual peak blood flow of the working muscle will be less than when a smaller muscle mass is involved. As convincingly developed by Rowell (1986), resistance of the active muscle during maximal aerobic exercise is reduced in a manner directed at controlling arterial blood pressure. Thus, during maximal aerobic exercise, such as cycling or running, the peak muscle blood flow is well below its vascular capacity and appears to be limited by the maximal cardiac output. This implies that an increase in muscle blood flow capacity is not necessary to achieve the increase in maximal aerobic capacity observed after training. An increase in maximal cardiac output could simply permit arterial pressure to be better maintained at a lower vascular resistance (and higher blood flow) of the active muscles. If the results of Saltin and co-workers (Andersen & Saltin, 1985; Rowell et al., 1986; Saltin, 1985) is applicable to mammalian skeletal muscle in general, then the training-induced increase in peak blood flow of working muscle during whole-body exercise (e.g., Musch et al., 1987) utilizes a greater fraction of the vascular reserve of the muscle. An increase in the capacity of the vascular circuit suggested by some data (Laughlin & Ripperger, 1987; Mackie & Terjung, 1983b) may not be an essential adaptation that occurs with exercise training.

Microvascular Changes in Muscle With Training

While blood flow to the active muscle is typically increased during maximal exercise after training, this is not the case during submaximal exercise. Blood flow to the active muscles working at a moderately intense exercise effort may actually be decreased slightly after training. An increased oxygen extraction of approximately 10% is often apparent across the working limb in trained individuals working at the same absolute power output as untrained individuals (cf. Clausen, 1976). Since oxygen consumption during this exercise effort is the same before and after training, blood flow to the active muscles should be slightly decreased. While the change in blood flow should be relatively small and difficult to measure, this expectation has been confirmed in some (cf. Clausen, 1976) but not all studies (e.g., Armstrong & Laughlin, 1984; Saltin et al., 1976). Further, since cardiac output is similar during the same submaximal work task before and after training, there should be an altered distribution of cardiac output to better perfuse noncontracting tissue. For example, a smaller reduction in splanchnic blood flow was found in trained animals during submaximal treadmill running (Armstrong & Laughlin, 1984). A smaller reduction in splanchnic blood flow is also typical of well-conditioned athletes with high aerobic capacities when working at the same absolute submaximal work rate (Rowell, 1986). Further, an increase in oxygen extraction during maximal aerobic exercise is typically observed after training, especially when the initial aerobic capacity of the individuals is relatively low (cf. Rowell, 1986). Thus, training-induced changes within the active muscle probably occur to optimize the exchange of oxygen.

Training induced increases in oxygen extraction by working muscle may be attributed to at least three factors. First, training increases the capillary density (cf. Gollnick & Saltin, 1982; Holloszy, 1973). Histochemically prepared cross sections of trained muscle typically exhibit a greater density of capillaries and a greater number of capillary contacts per muscle fiber. Perfusion of this greater capillary network could bring about a more effective distribution of blood flow within the muscle mass and account for the higher and more uniform pO_2 distribution found in trained muscle by Schroeder et al. (1976). The greater capillary surface area surrounding each fiber should also enhance nutrient exchange to better support the metabolic processes of the contracting muscle. Further, the enlarged capillary volume should help prolong RBC transit time for any given blood flow. This could be especially important during high flow conditions where the muscle energy flux and the demand for nutrient exchange is the greatest.

The second factor that could enhance oxygen extraction within muscle is an increase in mitochondrial content, which is typically found following exercise training (Gollnick & Saltin, 1982; Holloszy, 1973; Holloszy & Booth, 1976; Terjung & Hood, 1985). Evaluation of electron micrographs of trained muscle suggest that the greater content is due to both larger and more mitochondria (Gollnick & King, 1969). While this increase in mitochondrial density within the muscle fiber probably establishes important and beneficial changes in metabolic control during contractions (Dudley et al., 1987; Gollnick & Saltin, 1982; Holloszy, 1973; Holloszy & Booth, 1976), it could also serve to reduce the diffusion path length for oxygen (Sidell, 1983) and thereby contribute to a lower oxygen content in the muscle venous effluent.

Finally, an increase in muscle myoglobin concentration could also be beneficial for oxygen exchange. Myoglobin may be important during tissue oxygen exchange since it facilitates the diffusion of oxygen (Whittenberg, 1970) and probably accounts for the fairly uniform pO_2 throughout the cytosol of the fiber observed by Gayeski and Honig (1986). Thus, the increase in muscle myoglobin concentration induced by exercise training could reduce the resistance to oxygen exchange apparent between the sarcolemma and the mitochondrion. The overall benefit of these peripheral training adaptations has been demonstrated directly in studies where oxygen delivery to the contracting muscle of an isolated perfused rat hindlimb was high and the same for sedentary and trained muscles (Hood & Terjung, 1987; McAllister & Terjung, 1987). Muscle performance was better maintained, oxygen consumption was higher, and oxygen extraction was greater in the trained as compared to the sedentary group.

It is interesting to note that the capillary density (Gollnick & Saltin, 1982) and peak blood flow (Mackie & Terjung, 1983a) of a muscle section correlates well with the inherent oxidative capacity of the constituent muscle fibers. Different skeletal muscles (or fiber sections) appear to be "designed" in a manner that coordinates both the peak oxygen delivery and the microvascular system critical for oxygen exchange to the biochemical capacity of the tissue for aerobic metabolism (cf. Taylor et al., 1987). The results of Saltin and co-workers (Andersen & Saltin, 1985; Rowell et al., 1986; Saltin, 1985) are noteworthy in this regard. Their results of an extremely high oxygen uptake and muscle blood flow during single-limb knee extension exercise indicates that, even in untrained individuals, the "design" of muscle for oxidative metabolism possesses a capacity far greater than previously demonstrated. However, it appears likely that exercise training can induce adaptations within the muscle to further optimize aerobic function.

Physiological Significance of Muscle Vascular Changes

The physiological significance of a training-induced increase in peak muscle blood flow during maximal exercise is obvious. The greater oxygen delivery should lead to an increase in maximal oxygen consumption at a greater power output. This of course requires an increase in maximal cardiac output, since the redistribution of cardiac output during maximal exercise seems to be optimized even in the untrained state. As a result, perfusion of non-working tissues (e.g., splanchnic blood flow) during maximal exercise seems to be reduced similarly before and after exercise training (Musch et al., 1987). Thus, any significant increase in blood flow to the working muscle appears to require central cardiovascular adaptations to increase cardiac output. A further increase in maximal oxygen consumption in excess of that supported by the increase in cardiac output, however, can occur. An enhanced oxygen extraction, due to peripheral adaptations, can account for approximately 50% of the total training-induced increase in maximal oxygen consumption, especially when the subjects are initially relatively unfit (Rowell, 1986). Thus, a combination of central cardiovascular and peripheral adaptations can contribute to the increase in maximal aerobic work capacity often observed after exercise training.

The physiological significance of the fiber-type-specific changes observed in trained rats (Mackie & Terjung, 1983b) deserves consideration. Recall that an increase in apparent blood flow capacity was found in the fast-twitch white muscle section, but not in the fast-twitch red or slow-twitch red sections. If the 45% increase in maximal blood flow to the fast-twitch white muscle section were found in vivo, only a 10 to 15% increase in whole body maximal oxygen consumption would be expected. The overall quantitative effect of the increase in fast-twitch white section muscle blood flow would be significantly tempered by the fact that the relative blood flow to this muscle section is far below (approximately 1/4 to 1/3) the peak flows of the fast-twitch red muscle sections. Thus, most of the blood flow directed to the active muscles during exercise perfuses the richly vascularized high oxidative red type fibers (cf. Laughlin & Armstrong, 1985). If the peak blood flow to the red muscle sections did not increase with training, the increase in whole body maximal oxygen consumption with training would be fairly small and similar to that measured experimentally (Bedford et al., 1976; Patch & Brooks, 1980).

While the blood flow change in the fast-twitch white muscle may have limited impact on maximal aerobic capacity, this adaptation could contribute significantly to an improvement in endurance performance observed during fairly intense, but still submaximal, exercise after training. If an exercise intensity is chosen that cannot quite be sustained by recruiting only the red type fibers, then a small fraction of the fast-twitch white motor unit pool must be recruited. It is possible that this intensity of exercise may be excessive for many of the fast-twitch white motor units recruited prior to training but not afterwards. An increase in blood flow, coupled with an enriched capillary network surrounding the individual fast-twitch white fibers, may be just sufficient to increase their aerobic capacity by an amount necessary to better meet the energy demands of the contractile effort. The fast-twitch white motor units should perform better after training and thereby collectively contribute to a prolonged exercise duration. While this hypothesis remains to be supported by experimental evidence, it is consistent with the vastly improved endurance performance typically found after exercise training. Thus, it is likely that significant adaptations occur with training that impact on submaximal as well as maximal exercise conditions.

Acknowledgments

Work included from the authors' laboratory was supported by NIH grants AR 21617 and HL 37387.

References

Andersen, P., & Saltin, B. (1985). Maximal perfusion of skeletal muscle in man. *J. Physiol.*, **366**, 233-249.

Armstrong, R.B., & Laughlin, M.H. (1984). Exercise blood flow patterns within and among rat muscles after training. *Am. J. Physiol.*, **246**, H59-H68.

Bedford, T.G., Tipton, C.M., Wilson, N.C., Oppliger, R.A., & Gisolfi, C.V. (1976). Maximum oxygen consumption of rats and its change with various experimental procedures. *J. Appl. Physiol.*, **47**, 1278-1283.

Cerretelli, P., Marconi, C., Pendergast, D., Meyer, M., Heisler, N., & Piiper, J. (1984). Blood flow in exercising muscles by xenon clearance and by microsphere trapping. *J. Appl. Physiol.*, **56**, 24-30.

Clausen, J.P. (1976). Circulatory adjustments to dynamic exercise and effect of physical training in normal subjects and in patients with coronary artery disease. *Prog. In Cardiovasc. Dis.*, **38**, 459-495.

Dudley, G.A., Tullson, P.C., & Terjung, R.L. (1987). Influence of mitochondrial content on the sensitivity of respiratory control. *J. Biol. Chem*, **262**, 9109-9114.

Ekblom, B., & Hermansen, L. (1968). Cardiac output in athletes. *J. Appl. Physiol.*, **25**, 619-625.

Gayeski, T.E., & Honig, C.R. (1986). O_2 gradients from sarcolemma to cell interior in red muscle at maximal VO_2. *Am. J. Physiol.*, **251**, H789-H799.

Gollnick, P.D., & King, D.W. (1969). Effect of exercise training on mitochondria of rat skeletal muscles. *Am. J. Physiol.*, **216**, 1502-1509.

Gollnick, P.D., & Saltin, B. (1982). Significance of skeletal muscle oxidative enzyme enhancement with endurance training. *Clin. Physiol*, **2**, 1-12.

Holloszy, J.O. (1973). Biochemical adaptations to exercise: Aerobic metabolism. *Exer. and Sport Sci. Rev.*, **1**, 45-71.

Holloszy, J.O., & Booth, F.W. (1976). Biochemical adaptations to endurance exercise in muscle. *Ann. Rev. Physiol.*, **38**, 273-291.

Hood, D.A., Gorski, J., & Terjung, R.L. (1986). Oxygen cost of twitch and tetanic isometric contractions of rat skeletal muscle. *Am. J. Physiol.*, **250**, E449-E456.

Hood, D.A., & Terjung, R.L. (1987). Effect of endurance training on leucine metabolism in perfused rat skeletal muscle. *Am. J. Physiol.*, **253**, E648-E656.

Laughlin, M.H., & Armstrong, R.B. (1985). Muscle blood flow during locomotory exercise. *Ex. and Sport Sci. Rev.*, **13**, 95-136.

Laughlin, M.H., & Ripperger, J. (1987). Vascular transport capacity of hindlimb muscles of exercise trained rats. *J. Appl. Physiol.*, **62**, 438-443.

Mackie, B.G., & Terjung, R.L. (1983a). Muscle blood flows to the different fiber types during contraction. *Am. J. Physiol.*, **245**, H265-H275.

Mackie, B.G., & Terjung, R.L. (1983b). Influence of training on blood flow to different skeletal muscle fiber types. *J. Appl. Physiol.*, **55**, 1072-1078.

McAllister, R.M. & Terjung, R.L. (1987). Improved muscle performance due to peripheral adaptations induced by endurance training. *Med. Sci. Sports and Ex.*, **19**, S25.

Musch, T.I., Haidet, G.C., Ordway, G.A., Longhurst, J.C., & Mitchell, J.H. (1987). Training effects on regional blood flow response to maximal exercise in foxhounds. *J. Appl. Physiol.*, **62**, 1724-1732.

Patch, L.D., & Brooks, G.A. (1980). Effects of training on VO_2max and VO_2 during two running intensities in rats. *Pfluegers Arch.*, **386**, 215-219.

Rowell, L.B. (1986). *Human circulation: Regulation during physical stress.* New York, Oxford Univ. Press.

Rowell, L.B., Saltin, B., Kiens, B., & Christensen, N.J. (1986). Is peak quadriceps blood flow in humans even higher during exercise with hypoxemia? *Am. J. Physiol.*, **251**, H1038-H1044.

Saltin, B. (1985). Hemodynamic adaptations to exercise. *Am. J. Cardiol.*, **55**, 42D-47D.

Saltin, B., Nazar, K., Costill, D.L., Stein, E., Jannsson, E., Essen, B., & Gollnick, P.D. (1976). The nature of the training response: Peripheral and central adaptations to one-legged exercise. *Acta Physiol. Scand.*, **96**, 289-305.

Schroeder, W., Treumann, F., Ratscheck, W., & Muller, R. (1976). Muscle pO_2 in trained and untrained non-anesthetized guinea-pigs and in men. *Europ. J. Appl. Physiol.*, **351**, 215-221.

Sidell, B.D. (1983). Cellular acclimatization to environmental change by quantitative alterations in enzymes and organelles. In A.R. Cossins & R. Sheterline (Eds.), *Cellular acclimatization to environmental change.* Cambridge, Cambridge University Press, 103-120.

Snell, P.G., Martin, W.H., Buckey, J.C., & Blomqvist, C.G. (1987). Maximal vascular leg conductance in trained and untrained men. *J. Appl. Physiol.*, **62**, 606-610.

Taylor, C.R., Karas, R.H., Weibel, E.R., & Hoppeler, H. (1987). Adaptive variation in the mammalian respiratory system in relation to energetic demand. *Resp. Physiol.*, **69**, 1-127.

Terjung, R.L., & Hood, D.A. (1985). Biochemical adaptations in skeletal muscle induced exercise training. In D.K. Laymen (Ed.), *Nutrition and aerobic exercise.* Washington, DC: American Chemical Society, 8-26.

Wittenberg, J.A. (1970). Myoglobin-facilitated oxygen diffusion: Role of myoglobin in oxygen entry into muscle. *Physiol. Rev.*, **50**, 559-636.

Maximal Oxygen Uptake: Limitation and Malleability

B. Saltin

August Krogh Institute, University of Copenhagen, Copenhagen, Denmark

The aerobic capacity of man was once an essential component for survival. This is not the case today. Nevertheless, the interest in maximal oxygen uptake is still paramount. Its absolute magnitude and malleability with physical training has a bearing in sports. More important for the interest in the topic is probably that determination of oxygen uptake not only gives a measure of aerobic energy turnover, but also offers a precise measure of the capacity to transport and utilize oxygen. Thus, a good or high value for aerobic power indicates that the functional capacities of lungs, cardiovascular system, and muscle mitochondria are normal. Research in this field has been on-going for almost a century, and at regular intervals major reviews have been published (Åstrand, 1956; Blomqvist & Saltin, 1983; Christensen et al., 1934; Clausen, 1977; Rowell, 1974; Scheuer & Tipton, 1977). It could have been anticipated that a consensus had been reached on the most critical issue; namely, whether one factor in the chain of links of oxygen transport is limiting its utilization in the body. However, this is not the case. The views held at the present time are very far apart.

Weibel, Taylor, and associates have concluded that the limiting factor is the muscle mitochondria which all have to respire maximally to elicit maximal oxygen uptake (Taylor, 1987; Weibel, 1987). In line with this view is the finding of an increase in peak oxygen uptake only in the trained leg when one-legged training is performed (Saltin et al., 1976). The suggestion being that the local adaptations in the trained leg (i.e., increase in capillarity and mitochondrial enzyme level) are prerequisites for an elevation in peak oxygen uptake. In contrast a central limitation to maximal aerobic power is favored by many. Most commonly the pump capacity of the heart is pointed at (Ekblom, 1969; Rowell, 1987), but more lately have the lungs also come into focus (Dempsey et al., 1984). In this article the arguments for a central (heart) limitation of maximal oxygen uptake will be presented, as well as the role of the periphery (capillaries and mitochondrias) for endurance fitness. Further, the implication for performance and training will also be dwelt upon.

Pump Capacity of the Heart as a Limit to Maximal Aerobic Power

Early Studies

In the late 1920s and early 1930s Christensen proved that the heart rate response to exercise varied markedly between subjects, and that those performing regular physical activity usually could perform at a given submaximal work load with the lowest heart rate (Christensen, 1931). This observation prompted him to perform a longitudinal training study where a very substantial reduction in submaximal heart rate was achieved without an altered cardiac output (Figure 1). Thus, stroke volume became increased with the training. As the heart

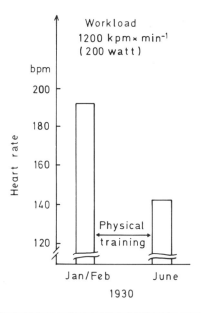

Figure 1. Redrawn from data published by Christensen (1931) in one subject (MN) who underwent endurance training. Heart rate was recorded during submaximal exercise, and cardiac output measurements revealed similar values (approximately 22-23 L • min⁻¹) in the two tests.

rate during exhaustive exercise was essentially the same regardless of training status, an elevated maximal cardiac output was suggested to be critical for improved aerobic work capacity.

These findings fell in line with the results of Henschen's ingenious studies (1899). By percutaneous percussion he estimated the size of the heart in cross-country skiers and found that the larger the heart the better the placing in the race. These findings, combined with equally classic findings on training rats (Petrow & Siebert, 1925; Siebert, 1929), formed the basis to point at the heart and its degree of hypertrophy as the key to success in endurance events. The rats were running with different speeds and durations on a treadmill. The results were clear. Intensity in endurance training was essential for an enlargement of the heart, and with that followed the best performance.

1950-1970

These two decades were the golden age for very elaborative studies of the central hemodynamics during exercise in humans. With the gain in experience during this period of placing catheters in various sections of the cardiovascular system, very detailed information was generated not only about systemic flow and its distribution, but also about the pressures necessary for perfusing the tissues and for an optimal filling of the ventricles of the heart (Bevegård & Shepherd, 1967; Holmgren & Åstrand, 1966; Wade & Bishop, 1962).

The most important findings were that the cardiac output linearly increased with exercise intensity (oxygen uptake) (Åstrand et al., 1964). Further, Christensen's findings were confirmed that maximal cardiac output varied with training status, which in turn was a function of the size of the stroke volume (Saltin et al., 1968). The regional distribution of the flow when going from rest to exercise was essentially unaltered to the brain (Ahlborg & Wahren, 1972), but was reduced in the kidneys in relation to the relative work load (Grimby, 1965), as well as in the splanchnic region (Rowell et al., 1968). This optimized the blood flow available for the heart and muscle and also allowed for an ample skin blood flow (Clausen, 1973). Mean arterial blood pressure became slightly elevated with the exercise with no apparent difference between untrained and trained subjects when exercise intensity was expressed in relative terms (Hartley et al., 1969). Central venous pressures as well as wedge pressure were also similar in well-trained and sedentary subjects (Bevegård et al., 1963; Granath & Strandell, 1964). The larger end-diastolic ventricular volumes associated with the large stroke volumes was then a function of less compliance of the ventricles of the trained men. Further, Henschen's early observation on the importance of the size of the heart was verified in a series of studies both in Scandinavia and in Germany (Reindell et al., 1957; Sjöstrand, 1955).

Longitudinal training studies produced results very similar to those observed in cross-sectional studies of persons with different physical training habits (Ekblom, 1969; Holmgren et al., 1960; Saltin et al., 1968). Thus, a quite firm conclusion could be made in regard to the effect of training on the circulation. The observations are summarized in Figure 2, where arterial oxygen delivery (x-axis) is related to the observed maximal oxygen uptake in a great number of studies. As the magnitude of the value on the x-axis is the product of maximal heart rate, stroke volume, and arterial oxygen content, and the first and last variables are almost unaffected by training, the stroke volume is the variable determining maximal oxygen delivery and thus the maximal oxygen uptake.

Further, support for delivery rather than utilization capacity being limiting was obtained from studies demonstrating an elevation in maximal oxygen uptake when oxygen-enriched

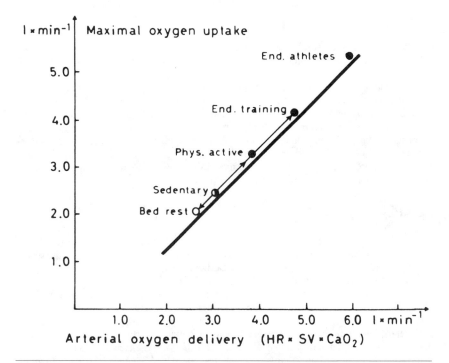

Figure 2.   Schematic summary of data in the literature (see text) on arterial delivery of oxygen and oxygen uptake during exhaustive (approximate 4-8 min) exercise (running or bicycling).

air was given during the exercise (Margaria et al., 1969) and when the exercise was performed at 3 ATM (Fagreus et al., 1973). Increasing the oxygen-carrying capacity of the blood by infusions of red cells also elevated the maximal oxygen uptake (Ekblom et al., 1972).

1970 to the Present

In 1968, Mellander and Johansson published a summary of the flow capacity of various organs and tissues of the body. They concluded that during maximal exercise the pump capacity of the heart could manage to supply most vascular beds of the body with an ample flow. This included the skeletal muscles which, when maximally vasodilatated, were thought to have a perfusion of 60 ml • 100 g^{-1} • min^{-1}. With 30 kg of muscle engaged in the exercise, 18 L • min^{-1} of flow were directed to the muscle and another 3 to 4 L • min^{-1} to other tissues and organs. This gave a maximal cardiac output of 21 to 22 L • min^{-1}, which was a very likely maximal value for a sedentary man weighing 70 to 80 kg.

What has been debated is whether peak perfusion of skeletal muscle in humans is "only" 60 ml • 100 g^{-1} • min^{-1} or whether this limit can be exceeded. In the past, plethysmography and later ^{133}Xe-washout curves have been used to establish peak perfusion of skeletal muscle, but both methods have limitations (Clausen, 1977; Snell et al., 1987). Lately a Doppler technique has been used to determine the velocity of the flow in the femoral artery, and estimations of blood flow have been made during intense rhythmic static contractions of the thigh muscles of one leg (Wesche, 1986). Mean muscle perfusion reached over 100 and peak flow above 200 ml • 100 g^{-1} • min^{-1} (Figure 3), without an elevation of mean

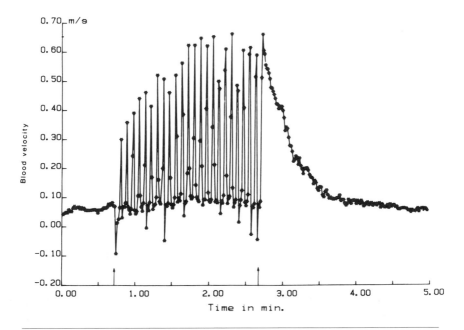

Figure 3.   Results from one subject performing intermittent static contractions with the knee-extensor muscles of one leg. Velocity of the blood flow in a. femoralis was measured with a Doppler technique (graph kindly produced by Wesche and Wallöe; Wesche, 1986).

arterial pressure. Similar or even higher values were obtained when one-legged dynamic knee extension was performed to exhaustion and blood flow was measured in the femoral vein using a constant infusion thermodilution method (Andersen & Saltin, 1985; Rowell et al., 1986; Table 1).

Critical to ascertaining a maximal muscle blood flow is that the work is performed with only a very small fraction of the muscle mass, as the central circulation seems to be a limiting link in oxygen transport. Further, as the number of capillaries and the oxidative potentials in various limb muscles of the body are not very large (Table 2), it appears safe to conclude that a large fraction of the muscle mass in humans has a perfusion capacity well above 60 ml • 100 g^{-1} • min^{-1}. The pump capacity of the heart cannot meet the demands of the contracting skeletal muscles for a flow when most of them are intensely recruited in exercise; that is, the capacity of skeletal muscles to receive a flow and consume the oxygen is much larger than what can be delivered to them, as the heart sets a ceiling when a critically large fraction of the muscle mass is engaged in the exercise.

Table 1 Mean Values (With SEM) for Some Variables Determined During Maximal Knee-Extensor Exercise With One Leg in 12 Healthy Subjects

Muscle mass (kg)	Oxygen uptake		Blood flow (L • min^{-1})	Mean arterial pressure (mmHg)
	Pulmonary (L • min^{-1})	Muscle (L • min^{-1})		
2.4	1.67	0.86	6.28	126
0.09	0.14	0.08	0.63	4

Table 2 Mean Values for Some Morphological Variables and a Mitochondrial Enzyme (Vmax) in Various Muscles of Sedentary Men

Muscle (man)	Slow twitch fibers (%)	Capillaries per mm^2	Citrate synthetase (μmoles • g^{-1} • min^{-1})
M. Soleus	89	390	7.6
M. Gastrocnemius	50	348	8.4
M. Quadriceps femoris, v.1	54	338	7.8
M. Trapezius	48	348	6.8
M. Deltoideus	52	308	7.9
M. Biceps brachii	42	374	9.4

Note. n = 6 to 15. A total of 15 subjects have been studied, with at least two different muscles examined in each subject.

General Considerations

In a way it can be said that the human body is not really designed for exercise using both upper and lower extremities simultaneously, at least not from the standpoint of the capacity of the heart as a pump. The system functions with the baroreceptors serving as the safety feedback. The sympathetic vasoconstrictor activity overrides any metabolic factors causing local vasodilatation, when the pump capacity of the heart is surpassed by the needs of the contracting muscles (Secher et al., 1977). The role of the sympathetic system is increased in relation to the fraction of the muscle mass involved in the exercise (Savard et al., 1989).

It would be interesting to be able to define in humans the mass of muscle which can be exercising intensely that can be supplied with a ''sufficient'' blood flow. Using the present data, it appears that in a sedentary person having a maximal cardiac output of 18 to 22 L • min⁻¹, 7 to 9 kg of muscle actively working could tax the capacity of the heart. Another way of expressing this would be to say that 1/4 to 1/3 of the total muscle mass of a sedentary person can consume 2.5 to 4.0 L • min⁻¹, or the equivalent to the maximal oxygen uptake of a sedentary person. In accordance with these estimates is the well-known fact that maximal oxygen uptake of a person is achieved in two-legged exercise (Bergh et al., 1976; Lewis et al., 1983; Table 3).

In an endurance athlete having a cardiac output of 30 to 40 L • min⁻¹ a larger muscle mass can be perfused reasonably well, but not maximally. This relates to rowing or swimming. If only the legs are intensely involved in the exercise, as in bicycling or running, they will obtain a larger flow and approach a maximal perfusion. As pointed out above, maximal vasodilatation cannot occur in all muscular beds at the same time maintaining normal blood pressure when two legs or more extremities perform the exercise. When a large fraction of the muscle mass is involved in the exercise, vasoconstriction must occur in vessels feeding contracting skeletal muscles. Indeed, this has been observed when arm work is added to leg exercise or when during one-legged exercise the other leg is included in the exercise (Klausen et al., 1982; Secher et al., 1977).

The above discussion does not deny that other limitations to oxygen transport and its consumption exist. The functional significances of these are, however, small. For example, the lungs at sea level already constitute a limitation (Dempsey et al., 1984; Terrados et al., 1985). If during exhaustive exercise alveolar oxygen tension was higher or an optimal transfer of oxygen could occur with a smaller alveolar–arterial O_2 gradient, more oxygen would be available in the arterial blood. Due to the shape of the hemoglobin–oxygen dissociation curve, the magnitude of such an elevation in arterial oxygen tension is marginal.

Table 3 Peak Oxygen Uptake and Cardiac Output During Exhaustive Exercise Performed With Different Fractions of the Muscle Mass

	Knee extensors (1 leg)	1 leg	2 legs	2 legs/2 arms
Variable				
Peak oxygen uptake (pulm.) L • min⁻¹	1.46	2.86	3.29	3.36
Peak cardiac output (L • min⁻¹)	10.5	18.4	19.9	20.5

Note. n = 3.

Similar evaluations can be made for each individual link in the oxygen transport, and it will be found that, from a functional standpoint, maximal oxygen delivery (maximal cardiac output • arterial oxygen content) is the variable that can vary the most and can thus be regarded as the most significant limitation to maximal oxygen uptake. This concept agrees well with the conclusion reached by Di Prampero (1985). He has approached this problem mathematically and estimated the relative role of each link in the oxygen transport.

Local Muscle Adaptation With Endurance Training: A Functional Significance?

Endurance training causes a proliferation of capillaries and elevation of the content of mitochondrial enzymes. It was first believed that these adaptations were a necessity for raising maximal oxygen uptake (see introduction). As this appears not to be the case, the pertinent question is what role these alterations in the muscle may have. The increased number of capillaries elevate capillary blood volume, which in turn means that at the same muscle blood flow mean transit time (MTT = capillary blood volume/muscle blood flow) is lengthened. This is not the only positive effect of more capillaries. As the capillary surface area is enlarged and if the increase in capillarization is larger than any increase in muscle fiber size, the area for diffusion is also smaller. All these factors contribute to improve the conditions of exchange between blood and muscle and will have some bearing on the extraction of oxygen, but its largest role is probably to make it possible to elevate the uptake of substrates (especially FFA) from the bloodstream.

With endurance training the metabolism during exercise is markedly altered. Respiratory exchange ratios (RER) are lower at a given work load and also at the same relative work load after endurance training, and the lactate production in muscle is reduced, which is reflected in a lower lactate level at a given absolute, but also at the same relative work load in the very well trained endurance athlete (Henriksson, 1977). This knowledge is not new. In the 1930s Bang (1936) made similar observations (Figure 4). What is new

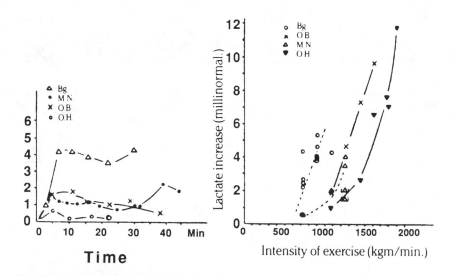

Figure 4.   The original drawing by Bang (1936). Blood lactate concentration is depicted at a given work load (left panel) and at different work loads (right panel) in four subjects in different training conditions.

is that we better understand how it is brought about. An attempt is made in Table 4 to present some of the factors that bring about the more efficient use of lipids as substrates for the muscle and concomitantly spates the glycogen breakdown. Of note is that more lipids or oxygen are not really offered to the trained muscles (Karlsson et al., 1972; Figure 5); rather it is the "quality" adaptations within the muscles that makes them superior in gearing the substrate choice from CHO to lipids and further saving the limited glycogen stores by a reduced rate of lactate formation. This is accomplished by careful control of the metabolism, which is improved in trained muscles (Gollnick & Saltin, 1982).

Table 4   List of Factors That Have a Bearing on the Regulation of Various Steps of the Muscle Metabolic Pathways

Variable	Trained	Untrained	Effect
ADP/ATP	Low	High	Activates PFK
Cytoplasmatic FA	High	Low	Inhibits PFK
Mitochondrial FA	High	Low	a) Inhibits PDH b) Increased flux through through β-oxidation
Cytoplasmatic citrate	High	Low	Inhibits PFK

Note. A comparison is made between endurance-trained and untrained muscles. A high ADP/ATP ratio activates phosphofructokinase (PFK). High concentrations of fatty acids (FA) inhibit PFK and, in the mitochondria, pyruvate dehydrogenase, whereas the β-oxidation is increased. A high citrate concentration has been proposed to inhibit PFK.

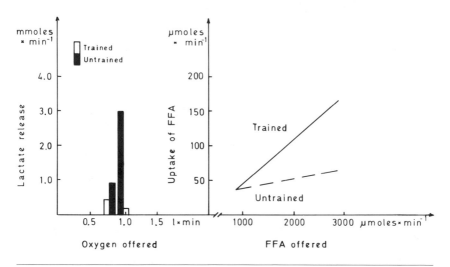

Figure 5. Summary of data from a one-legged training study where to the left is depicted the volume of oxygen delivered to the trained and untrained limb, respectively, and the lactate release. To the right is similar data on amount of FFA offered and the uptake of FFA by trained and untrained muscles (Henriksson, 1977; Kiens et al., 1989).

Practical Implications

One important practical implication of the above discussed findings is that training of endurance can be divided into two components aiming at the improvement of the pump capacity of the heart, which is then closely related to the maximal oxygen uptake of the subject. The peripheral adaptation with increased capillarization and elevated oxidative potential in the muscles is the other component whose functional significance mainly is to optimize substrate utilization of the muscle and thereby improve endurance capacity.

This dissociation between maximal oxygen uptake and muscle adaptation for performance has been nicely demonstrated experimentally. If road runners stop their training for two weeks, maximal oxygen uptake only drops by 2 to 3%, but performance measured as the time to exhaustion at a given speed was reduced by 24% (Houston et al., 1979; Figure 6). Incidentally there was also a reduction in the oxidative capacity of the muscle of the same magnitude as in performance. Recently Coyle et al. (1986) have added to this and demonstrated that the reduction in maximal oxygen uptake, although small, is reversible by expanding the plasma volume, which in turn made the short-term work performance (4 min) return to pre-detraining level.

Another example can be taken from the preparation for the Tour de France (Sjøgaard et al., 1982). When the bicyclists were studied in February they had a maximal oxygen uptake of 74 ml • kg^{-1} • min^{-1}, which was only increased by 5% over the five months of intensive training up to the start of the Tour de France in July (Table 5). Oxidative enzymes in the limb muscles, on the other hand, doubled during the same time period, resulting in a four-fold higher mitochondrial enzyme level in these bicyclists than found in muscle of sedentary men, an adaptation most needed for optimal fuel economy during such a long race.

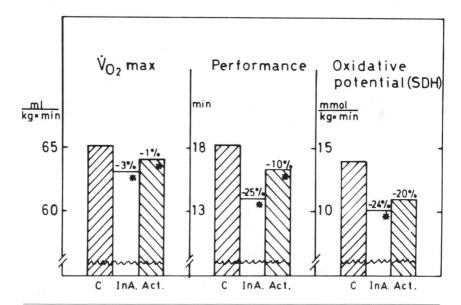

Figure 6. Data on well-trained road runners (n = 6), who stopped all training for 2 weeks and then resumed the training. Measurements of maximal oxygen uptake (VO$_2$max) on the treadmill, time to exhaustion, and an oxidative enzyme (succinate dehydrogenase = SDH) were performed when in top condition (C), after 14 days of inactivity (in A), and after training had been resumed for 14 days (Act) (Houston et al., 1979).

Table 5 Maximal Oxygen Uptake and Some Mitochondrial Enzymes in a Limb Muscle of Professional Bicyclists

	Professional bicyclists	
	February	July
$\dot{V}O_2$max (ml • kg^{-1} • min^{-1})	74	77
Enzymes:		
CS (mmoles • kg^{-1} • min^{-1} d.w.)	69	112
HAD (mmoles • kg^{-1} • min^{-1} d.w.)	66	104

Note. Based on data obtained at the start of systematic preparation for the season and one week before the Tour de France (July). From Sjøgaard et al., 1982.

Another implication of the above results relates to an optimal training pattern of the heart. It is apparent that a minimum muscle mass must be involved in the exercise to train the heart. One-legged training (7-8 kg muscle) is not sufficient even if the training sessions are quite long (Saltin et al., 1976) or repeated with each leg (Klausen et al., 1982). Two-legged exercise is a minimum, but whether the inclusion of arm work or performing in a supine position improve the training stimulus is not known. Rowers and cross-country skiers have the very highest reported values for maximal oxygen uptake (in L • min^{-1} approximately 7.50; in ml • kg^{-1} • min^{-1} approximately 90). It is of note, however, that these high values can be achieved when the athletes exercise only with their legs, running (Bergh, 1974; Secher, 1983).

Detraining—Retraining

A myth is that if you have trained once and achieved a good capacity, it is easier to return to the same level if, for one reason or another, you have been away from regular training for some time. This is not true and has been demonstrated for sedentary people undergoing training (Figure 7; Pedersen & Jørgensen, 1978) as well as for formerly very successful athletes (Eriksson et al., 1975). It is true that dimensions of the lungs and the heart do not change so rapidly (Rost & Hollman, 1983). Of greater importance is, however, that the functional capacity relates to quality of the various organs or tissues. The content of enzymes in a tissue or the degree of capillarization of skeletal muscle do change more rapidly than the volume or size of a tissue or organ (Booth, 1977; Henriksson & Reitman, 1977; Klausen et al., 1981). Possible time constants for a change in certain variables to occur are given in Table 6.

The size of the heart develops slowly (Rost & Hollman, 1983). Elovanio and Sundberg (1983) found no difference in the 14-year-old between runners (with at least 2 years of endurance training) and controls, but in a follow-up study after 5 years a clear-cut difference was observed. In adults faster changes have been seen, but the changes in the heart size must be regarded as rather slow. Blood volume is changed faster than the heart size, but it is dependent upon the dimensional development of the cardiovascular system for an optimal adaptation. The alterations that take place in muscle can occur quite fast if the optimal stimulus (training pattern) is present. If it is removed the return to control level goes fast (Booth, 1977). Capillary proliferation or reduction can occur with a time constant of weeks (Andersen & Henriksson, 1977; Klausen et al., 1981), which is slightly lower than the mitochondrial enzymes (Henriksson & Reitman, 1977).

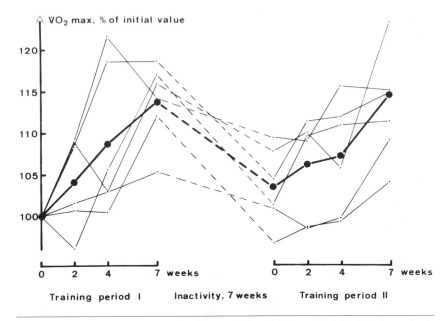

Figure 7. Young healthy sedentary females were followed. They trained for 7 weeks on fixed loads and times on bicycle ergometers. Thereafter no training was performed for 7 weeks. Identical training as during the first period was again performed. Individual and mean values for maximal oxygen uptake are given (Pedersen & Jørgensen, 1978).

Table 6   Summary of Approximate Times for an Adaptation to Occur

Variable	Time for a change
Heart size	Months - years
Plasma volume	Weeks
Red cell volume	Months
Skeletal muscle capillaries	Weeks - months
Skeletal muscle mitochondrial enzymes	Weeks

Based on the information given in Table 6 it can be said that to improve the pump capacity of the heart (= maximal oxygen uptake) there is a need for training over a long period of time (years). Muscle capillaries and oxidative enzymes can be brought to quite high levels with regular training lasting 6 to 12 months. As it always takes a longer time to elevate an enzyme or a capacity than it takes to lose the adaptation, it must be of value to maintain some regularity in training with a few training sessions also in the period between seasons.

To conclude, it can be stated that the primary factors setting the athlete's pace in an endurance event are maximal oxygen uptake and technique (energy costs for a given speed).

The time this speed can be maintained is a function of efficiency in fuel utilization (glycogen swing) and glycogen storage in the body (muscle/liver). These factors set the relative work rate and how long the speed can be maintained (Table 7).

Table 7 Summary of the Factors That Set the Pace and Determine the Duration This Pace Can be Maintained

Endurance exercise

Speed (work rate)	Maximal oxygen uptake
	Efficiency (technique)
Duration (maintain speed at a high relative work rate [% of $\dot{V}O_2max$])	Efficiency in usage of CHO ("glycogen saving"); glycogen stores

Acknowledgments

The research performed in our own laboratory was supported by grants from the Danish Heart Foundation and the Research Council of the Danish Sport Federation.

References

Ahlborg, G., & Wahren, J. (1972). Brain substrate utilization during prolonged exercise. *Scandinavian Journal of Clinical Laboratory Investigation, 29*, 397-402.

Anderson, P., & Henriksson, J. (1977). Capillary supply of the quadriceps femoris muscle of man: Adaptive response to exercise. *Journal of Physiology (London), 270*, 677-690.

Andersen, P., & Saltin, B. (1985). Maximal perfusion of skeletal muscle in man. *Journal of Physiology (London), 366*, 233-249.

Åstrand, P.-O. (1956). Human physical fitness with special reference to sex and age. *Physiological Review, 6*, 307.

Åstrand, P.-O., Cuddy, T.E., Saltin, B., & Stenberg, J. (1964). Cardiac output during submaximal and maximal work. *Journal of Applied Physiology, 19*, 268-274.

Bang, O. (1936). The lactate content of the blood during and after muscular exercise in man. *Scandinavisches Archive für Physiologie, 74(10)*, 51-82.

Bergh, U. (1974). *"Längdlöpning," Idrottsfysiologi, rapport no. 11*. Trygg-Hansa, Stockholm (in Swedish).

Bergh, U., Kanstrup, I.-L., & Ekblom, B. (1976). Maximal oxygen uptake during exercise with various combinations of arm and leg work. *Journal of Applied Physiology, 41*, 191-196.

Bevegård, S., Holmgren, A., & Jonsson, B. (1963). Circulatory studies in well trained athletes at rest and during heavy exercise, with special reference to stroke volume and the influence of body position. *Acta Physiologica Scandinavica, 57*, 26-50.

Bevegård, B.S., & Shepherd, J.T. (1967). Regulation of the circulation during exercise in man. *Physiological Review, 47*, 178-213.

Blomqvist, C.G., & Saltin, B. (1983). Cardiovascular adaptations to physical training. *Annual Review of Physiology, 45*, 69-89.

Booth, F.W. (1977). Effects of endurance exercise on cytochrome C turnover in skeletal muscle. *Annals New York Academy of Sciences, 3*, 431-400.

Christensen, E.H. (1931). Beitrage zur Physiologie schwerer körperlicher. IV: Mitteilung: Die Pulsfrequenz während und unmittelbar nach schwerer körperlicher Arbeit. *Arbeits Physiologie*, **4**, 453-469.

Christensen, E.H., Krogh, A., & Lindhard, J. (1935). Investigations on heavy muscular work. *Quarterly Bulletin on the Health Organisation of the League of Nations*, **3**, 388.

Clausen, J.P. (1973). Muscle blood flow during exercise and its significance for maximal performance. In J. Keul (Ed.), *Limiting factors of physical performance*, Stuttgart, Georg Thieme, 253.

Clausen, J.P. (1977). Effect of physical training on cardiovascular adjustments to exercise in man. *Physiological Review*, **57**, 779-815.

Coyle, E.F., Hemmert, M.K., & Coggan, A.R. (1986). Effects of detraining on cardiovascular responses to exercise: Role of blood volume. *Journal of Applied Physiology*, **60(1)**, 95-99.

Dempsey, J.A., Hanson, P., & Henderson, K. (1984). Exercise-induced arterial hypoxemia in healthy humans at sea-level. *Journal of Physiology (London)*, **355**, 161-175.

Di Prampero, P. (1985). Metabolic and circulatory limitations to VO_2max at the whole animal level. *Journal of Experimental Biology*, **115**, 319-331.

Ekblom, B. (1969). Effect of physical training on oxygen transport system in man. *Acta Physiologica Scandinavica*, (Suppl. 328), 5-45.

Ekblom, B., Goldberg, A.N., & Gullbring, B. (1972). Response to exercise after blood loss and reinfusion. *Journal of Applied Physiology*, **33**, 175-180.

Elovainio, R., & Sundberg, S. (1983). A five-year follow-up study on cardiorespiratory function in adolescent elite endurance runners. *Acta Paediatrica Scandinavica*, **72**, 351-356.

Eriksson, B.O., Lundin, A., & Saltin, B. (1975). Cardiopulmonary function in former girl swimmers and the effects of physical training. *Scandinavian Journal of Clinical and Laboratory Investigation*, **35**, 135.

Fagreus, L., Karlsson, J., Linnarsson, D., & Saltin, B. (1973). Oxygen uptake during maximal work at lowered and raised ambient air pressures. *Acta Physiologica Scandinavica*, **87**, 411-421.

Gollnick, P.D. & Saltin, B. (1982). Significance of skeletal muscle oxidative enzyme enhancement with endurance training. *Clinical Physiology*, **2**, 1-12.

Granath, A., & Strandell, T. (1964). Relationships between cardiac output, stroke volume and intracardiac pressures at rest and during exercise in supine position and some anthropometric data in healthy old men. *Acta Medica Scandinavica*, (Suppl. 414).

Grimby, G. (1965). Renal clearances during prolonged supine exercise at different loads. *Journal of Applied Physiology*, **20**, 1264.

Hartley, L.H., Grimby, G., Kilbom, Å., et al. (1969). Physical training in sedentary middle-aged and older men. *Scandinavian Journal of Clinical and Laboratory Investigation*, **24**, 335.

Henriksson, J. (1977). Training induced adaptation of skeletal muscle and metabolism during submaximal exercise. *Journal of Physiology (London)*, **270**, 661-674.

Henriksson, J., & Reitman, J.S. (1977). Time course of changes in human skeletal muscle succinate dehydrogenase and cytochrome oxidase activities and maximal oxygen uptake with physical activity and inactivity. *Acta Physiologica Scandinavica*, **99**, 91-97.

Henschen, E.S. (1899). *Skidlauf und Skidwettlauf. Eine medizinische Sportsstudie.* Mitteilungen Medicinische Klinik, Uppsala, Jena Fischer Verlag.

Holmgren, A., Mossfeldt, F., Sjöstrand, T., et al. (1960). Effect of training on work capacity, total hemoglobin, blood volume, heart volume, and pulse rate in recumbent and upright positions. *Acta Physiologica Scandinavica*, **50**, 72.

Holmgren, A., Åstrand, P.-O. (1966). D_L and the dimensions and functional capacities of the O_2 transport system in humans. *Journal of Applied Physiology*, **21**, 1463-1470.

Houston, M.E., Bentzen, H., & Larsen, H. (1979). Interrelationships between skeletal muscle adaptations and performance as studied by detraining and retraining. *Acta Physiologica Scandinavica*, **105**, 163-170.

Karlsson, J., Nordesjö, L.-O., Jorfeldt, L., & Saltin, B. (1972). Muscle lactate, ATP and CP levels during exercise after physical training in man. *Journal of Applied Physiology*, **33**, 199-203.

Klausen, K., Andersen, L.B., & Pelle, I. (1981). Adaptive changes in work capacity, skeletal muscle capillarization and enzyme levels during training and detraining. *Acta Physiologica Scandinavica*, **113**, 9-16.

Klausen, K., Secher, N.G., Clausen, P., Hartling, O., & Trap-Jensen, J. (1982). Central and regional circulatory adaptations to one-legged training. *Journal of Applied Physiology: Respirat. Environ. Exer. Physiol.*, **52**, 976-983.

Lewis, S.F., Taylor, W.F., Graham, R.M., Pettinger, W.A., Schutter, J.E., & Blomqvist, C.G. (1983). Cardiovascular responses to exercise as functions of absolute and relative work load. *Journal of Applied Physiology*, **54**, 1314-1323.

Margaria, R., Cerretelli, P., Marchi, S., & Rossi, L. (1969). Maximum exercise in oxygen. *Internationales Zeitschrift Angewandte Physiologie*, **18**, 465-467.

Mellander, S., & Johansson, B. (1968). Control of resistance, exchange, and capacitance functions in the peripheral circulation. *Pharmacological Reviews*, **20**, 117.

Pedersen, P.K., & Jørgensen, K. (1978). Maximal oxygen uptake in young women with training, inactivity, and retraining. *Medicine and Science in Sport*, **10(4)**, 233-237.

Petrow, H., & Siebert, W. (1925). Studien über Arbeitshypertrophie des Muskels. *Zeitschrift für Klinische Medizin*, **102**, 428-433.

Reindell, H., Klepzig, H., Musshoff, K., Kirchhoff, H.W., Steim, H., Moser, F., & Frisch, P. (1957). Neuere Untersuchungsergebnisse über Beziehungen zwischen Grösse und Leistungsbreite des gesunden menschlichen Herzens, insbesondere des Sportherzens. *Deutsche Medicinische Wochenschrift*, **82**, 613-619.

Roskamm, H. (1971). Central circulatory adjustment to exercise in well-trained subjects. In O.A. Larsen & O. Malmborg (Eds.), *Coronary heart disease and physical fitness*. Copenhagen, Munksgaard, 17.

Rost, R., & Hollmann, W. (1983). Athlete's heart—A review of its historical assessment and new aspects. *International Journal of Sports Medicine*, **4**, 147-165.

Rowell, L.B., Brengelmann, G.L., Blackmon, J.R., Twiss, R.D., & Kusumi, F. (1968). Splanchnic blood flow and metabolism in heat-stressed humans. *Journal of Applied Physiology*, **24**, 475-484.

Rowell, L.B. (1974). Cardiovascular adjustments to exercise and thermal stress. *Physiological Reviews*, **54**, 75-159.

Rowell, L.B., Saltin, B., Kiens, B., & Christensen, N.J. (1986). Is peak quadriceps blood flow in humans even higher during exercise with hypoxemia? *American Journal of Physiology*, **251**, H1038-H1044.

Saltin, B., Blomqvist, G., Mitchell, J.H., Johnson, R.L. Jr., Wildenthal, K., & Chapman, C.B. (1968). Response to exercise after bed rest and after training. *Circulation*, **38(7)**, 1-78.

Saltin, B., Nazar, K., Costill, P.L., Stein, E., Jansson, E., Essen, B., & Gollnick, P.D. (1976). The nature of the training response: Peripheral and central adaptations to one-legged exercise. *Acta Physiologica Scandinavica*, **96**, 289-305.

Savard, G.K., Richter, E.A., Strange, S., Kiens, B., Christensen, N.J., & Saltin, B. (1989). Norepinephrine spillover from skeletal muscle during dynamic exercise in man: Role of muscle mass. *American Journal of Physiology*. In press.

Scheuer, J., & Tipton, C.M. (1977). Cardiovascular adaptations to physical training. *Annual Review of Physiology*, **39**, 221-251.

Secher, N.H., Clausen, J.P., Klausen, K., Nore, I., & Trap-Jensen, J. (1977). Central and regional circulatory effects of adding arm exercise to leg exercise. *Acta Physiologica Scandinavica*, **100**, 288-297.

Secher, N.H. (1983). The physiology of rowing. *Journal of Sports Sciences*, **1**, 23.

Siebert, W. (1929). Untersuchungen über Hypertrophie des Skeletmuskels. *Zeitschrift für Klinische Medizin*, **109**, 350-354.

Sjøgaard, G., Nielsen, B., Mikkelsen, F., & Saltin, B. (1982). Etude physiologique du cyclisme. *Colloques Medico-Sportifs de Saint-Etienne*.

Sjöstrand, T. (1955). Das Sportherz. *Arzt und Sport*, **80**, 963-966.

Snell, P.G., Martin, W.H., Buckey, J.C., & Blomqvist, C.G. (1987). Maximal vascular leg conductance in trained and untrained men. *Journal of Applied Physiology*, **62**, 606-610.

Taylor, C.R. (1987). Structural and functional limits to oxidative metabolism: Insights from scaling. *Annual Review of Physiology*, **49**, 135-146.

Terrados, N., Mizuno, M., & Andersen, H. (1985). Reduction in maximal oxygen uptake at low altitudes: Role of training status and lung function. *Clinical Physiology*, **5(3)**, 75-79.

Wade, O.L., & Bishop, J.M. (1962). *Cardiac output and regional blood flow*. Oxford, Blackwell.

Weibel, E.R. (1987). Scaling of structural and functional variables in the respiratory system. *Annual Review of Physiology*, **49**, 147-159.

Wesche, J. (1986). The time course and magnitude of blood flow changes in the human quadriceps muscles following isometric contraction. *Journal of Physiology*, **44**, 151-164.

Calcium Shifts and Force–Frequency Relations in Heart Muscle and the Origin of Activator Calcium in Postrest Potentiation in Atria

A. Prokopczuk

Postgraduate Center of Medical Education, Warsaw, Poland

Contractile force (CF) of the heart muscle largely depends on the rate and pattern of stimulation (Koch-Weser & Blinks, 1963). The response of the myocardial CF to the rate of steady-state stimulation is called the force–frequency relation. Its extreme forms are rest decay and postrest recovery of CF. Recently, Capogrossi et al. (1986) have shown that the force–frequency relation is a property of single isolated cardiac myocytes. Force–frequency relation seems to be the most intrinsic of the heart mechanisms for the control of its strength. The rate of stimulation has been proved to affect the transmembrane Ca^{2+} fluxes and cellular Ca^{2+} content (Bers & MacLeod, 1986; Chapman & Niedergerke, 1970; Langer, 1965).

The activation-dependent Ca^{2+} exchange has been for the last several years the area of our investigations. We found (Pytkowski et al., 1983) that beat-to-beat Ca^{2+} influx is inversely related to the rate of steady-state stimulation and to CF, as well as to the CF during postrest recovery. Voltage clamp experiments demonstrated decreases of calcium current during positive rate staircases (Simurda et al., 1981). These results suggest that CF developed in response to the excitation-dependent calcium influx may be primed by some intracellular factor.

On the basis of our experiments, we proposed (Pytkowski et al., 1983) that in guinea pig ventricular muscle there are two intracellular fractions of exchangeable calcium: (a) fraction exchanged from beat-to-beat, which we labeled after Chapman and Niedergerke (1970) Ca_1, and (b) the second fraction named Ca_2, which is hardly exchangeable under conditions of steady-state stimulations, but is completely lost from the cells during prolonged rest and recovered during postrest (PR) stimulation. Its Ca^{2+} content is positively and linearly correlated with CF during both rest decay and PR recovery, and it changes linearly with the stimulation rate between 0.45 ± 0.05 (resting value) and 1.65 ± 0.12 mmol • kg^{-1} wet weight (w.w.) (Lewartowski et al., 1984). On this basis we suggested that Ca_2 may constitute an important component of the mechanism of force–frequency relations.

Such an assumption has found its rationale in comparative studies in various species. Fraction Ca_2 is large (about 1.0 mmol • kg^{-1} w.w.) in guinea pig ventricles, which display a positive staircase in response to PR stimulation and deep rest decay (Pytkowski et al., 1983); it is smaller in rabbit ventricles (about 0.35 mmol • kg^{-1} w.w.), and negligible in rat (about 0.1 mmol • kg^{-1} w.w.) (Janczewski & Lewartowski, 1986). Rabbit ventricles reveal a positive staircase and rest decay; however, the rate of postrest recovery is twice as high as in the guinea pig ventricles. Contrary to other species investigated, rat ventricles show a negative staircase and no rest decay. Hence, the results of comparative studies clearly show that differences in the pattern of response of CF to the prolonged rest between various species find their counterpart in the respective differences in the pattern of rest- and stimulation-dependent shifts of the tissue Ca^{2+}, which is consistent with the proposed hypothesis. It further applies to the differences between various parts of the heart.

In guinea pig atria the first postrest contraction (PRC) is greatly potentiated, and, as reported previously (Prokopczuk, 1987; Prokopczuk & Lewartowski, 1985) Ca_2 fraction is present in this part of the heart. It was proposed (Prokopczuk, 1987) that release of Ca^{2+} from Ca_2 during rest in atria primes with Ca^{2+} calcium pool supporting the potentiated PRC. This pool, commonly assumed to be localized in the sarcoplasmic reticulum (SR) (Chapman, 1983; Manning & Hollander, 1971) does not seem to be identical with Ca_2 pool. If so, then a question arises as to the subcellular localization of Ca_2 fraction. To solve this problem further, an attempt was made to block selectively the release of Ca^{2+} from the SR and to observe the remaining intracellular Ca^{2+} after rest, as well as to modify mitochondrial Ca^{2+} fluxes. Description of technical set up and measurement of $^{45}Ca^{2+}$ content is given in detail elsewhere (Prokopczuk, 1987; Prokopczuk & Lewartowski, 1985; Pytkowski et al., 1983). Briefly, calcium uptake was estimated as $^{45}Ca^{2+}$ uptake under conditions of full equilibration of the preparations with $^{45}Ca^{2+}$, that is, after incubation with $^{45}Ca^{2+}$ for 60 min while paced at 1 Hz. Cellular $^{45}Ca^{2+}$ content was calculated by subtracting the estimated content of free $^{45}Ca^{2+}$ within the extracellular space from the total tissue $^{45}Ca^{2+}$ content, and the extracellular space was measured by means of $^{35}SO_4^{2-}$. Isometric contractions were recorded in some experiments at L_{max} (the length at which maximal CF is developed). Two chemical agents were applied: caffeine in a concentration of 12.5 mmol, and carbonyl cyanide m-chlorophenyl hydrazone (CCCP) in a concentration of 2 μmol.

It was found previously (Prokopczuk, 1987) that in guinea pig atria a 10-min rest caused a drop in $^{45}Ca^{2+}$ content from 3.79 $\pm$ 0.14 to 3.01 $\pm$ 0.07 mmol • kg^{-1} w.w. (Table 1, column 1, rows 1 and 2). When three PR beats were introduced, the first PRC was strongly potentiated, whereas there was a large net loss of Ca^{2+}, as $^{45}Ca^{2+}$ content decreased further to 2.50 $\pm$ 0.14 mmol • kg^{-1} w.w. (Table 1, column 1, row 3), presumably mostly during the first contraction. It should be noted that this finding has recently been confirmed by Hilgemann (1986a, 1986b) who, using a different experimental approach (measurement of extracellular calcium with tetramethylmurexide), found depletion of Ca^{2+} from the cell by the PR excitations.

Subsequent stimulation for the next 10 min resulted in a full recovery of CF and $^{45}Ca^{2+}$ content (Prokopczuk, 1987; Prokopczuk & Lewartowski, 1985). Caffeine (12.5 mmol) applied at the beginning of a 10-min rest period abolished potentiation of the first PRC and augmented the steady-state CF by about 50% $\pm$ 25% (Figure 1). Under the conditions of steady-state stimulation caffeine did not alter $^{45}Ca^{2+}$ uptake (Table 1, column 2, row 1). It did not either influence the magnitude of a drop in $^{45}Ca^{2+}$ content following the 10-min

Table 1   Effects of Caffeine (12.5 mmol) and CCCP (2 μmol) Applied for the Last 10 Min of Exposure to $^{45}CA^{2+}$ on the $^{45}Ca^{2+}$ Content (mmol/kg w.w.; Means $\pm$ SD; n = 7-10) in Guinea Pig Atria Under Various Stimulation Patterns

Stimulation pattern	Control	Caffeine	CCCP	Caffeine + CCCP
55 min stim.	3.79 $\pm$ 0.14	3.88 $\pm$ 0.18	3.74 $\pm$ 0.24	2.44 $\pm$ 0.18
45 min stim. + 10-min rest	3.01 $\pm$ 0.07	2.96 $\pm$ 0.21	3.12 $\pm$ 0.19	2.38 $\pm$ 0.21
45 min stim. + 10-min rest + 3 postrest excitations	2.50 $\pm$ 0.14	2.85 $\pm$ 0.18	3.01 $\pm$ 0.2	2.41 $\pm$ 0.23

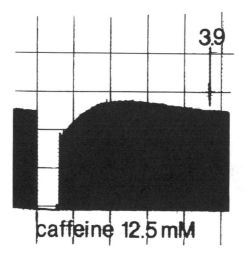

Figure 1. Effects of caffeine (12.5 mmol) on postrest recovery of contractile force and $^{45}Ca^{2+}$ content in guinea pig atrium after a 10-min rest.

rest. Three subsequent excitations evoked after rest under these circumstances had no additional effect, contrary to the control conditions (Table 1, column 2, rows 2 & 3).

Exposure to CCCP at the beginning of a 10-min rest diminished markedly the first PRC (Figure 2a) and abolished steady-state contractions inducing a slight contracture (Figure 2b); however, rather unexpectedly, it produced no detectable change in $^{45}Ca^{2+}$ content in steady-state conditions (Table 1, column 3, row 1). Likewise, addition of CCCP to the perfusate at the beginning of the 10-min rest caused no significant alteration in $^{45}Ca^{2+}$ content comparing with control (3.12 ± 0.19 and 3.01 ± 0.07 mmol · kg^{-1} w.w., respectively). This time the postrest content also failed to be affected by the three postrest excitations (Table 1, column 1, rows 2 & 3). When caffeine and CCCP were applied together, steady-state contractions were abolished and a contracture of about 200% of previously recorded phasic contractions developed (Figure 3). Simultaneous exposure to both agents caused a decrease of $^{45}Ca^{2+}$ to 2.44 ± 0.18 mmol · kg^{-1} w.w. (Table 1, column 4, row 1). No further alterations in $^{45}Ca^{2+}$ content were observed after rest and postrest excitations (Table 1, column 4, rows 2 & 3).

In the present study Ca^{2+} distribution in atrial myocardium was examined under various Ca^{2+} loading conditions using caffeine as a probe for determination of involvement of the SR in Ca^{2+} exchange, and CCCP to study mitochondrial Ca^{2+} exchange (Langer & Nudd, 1980; Lehninger et al., 1978).

Both caffeine and CCCP applied separately had seemingly no effect on $^{45}Ca^{2+}$ content in guinea pig atria, regardless of whether it was steady-state stimulation or rest or postrest excitations, at which they exerted analogous influence giving no further changes in $^{45}Ca^{2+}$ content established after the 10-min rest, although the respective contractile responses were so much at variance.

Caffeine was found to decrease the rate of SR calcium uptake and stimulate SR calcium release (Rasmussen et al., 1987; Takashima et al., 1980; Weber & Herz, 1968). Thus, a significant decrease in fraction Ca_2 could be expected under exposure to caffeine if Ca_2 were localized in the SR. However, it was not the case. As it was found in our laboratory, mitochondrial uncoupler protonofore CCCP displaced fraction Ca_2 from the guinea pig ventricular myocardium nearly completely, and partially from the rat ventricular muscle

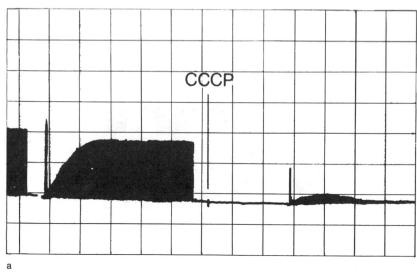

a

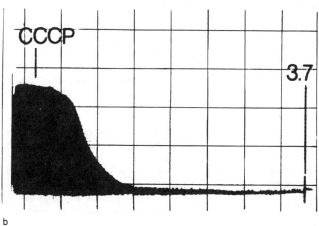

b

Figure 2.   Effects of CCCP (2 μmol) on (a) postrest recovery of contractile force in guinea pig atrium after a 10-min rest; (b) contractile force and $^{45}Ca^{2+}$ content in guinea pig atrium stimulated at a rate 1 Hz.

(Janczewski & Lewartowski, 1986), which suggests mitochondria as a possible Ca_2 site. Nevertheless, in the guinea pig atrial tissue CCCP alone did not augment $^{45}Ca^{2+}$ loss during rest and PR stimulation. Only when caffeine and CCCP were applied together was the $^{45}Ca^{2+}$ content lowered to the resting level under all stimulation patterns. This indicates that Ca^{2+} defined as Ca_2 fraction cycles between these two compartments: SR and mitochondria, and both of them play a significant role in contractile Ca^{2+} exchange of the cells. Ca^{2+} released from mitochondria by CCCP may be sequestered by the SR, and vice versa: Ca^{2+} released by caffeine from the SR may be taken up by mitochondria. Effective inhibition of both compartments by simultaneous application of these two agents blocks uptake of

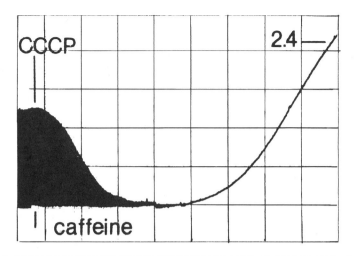

Figure 3. Effects of simultaneous application of caffeine (12.5 mmol) and CCCP (2 μmol) on contractile force and $^{45}Ca^{2+}$ content in guinea pig atrium stimulated at a rate 1 Hz.

Ca^{2+} by organelle in question, resulting in Ca^{2+} release into the sarcoplasma, as evidenced by contracture, and is subsequently followed by Ca^{2+} extrusion from the cell. Recent evidence shows that the first PRC is mostly dependent on intracellular calcium stores (Bers, 1983, 1985).

The presented findings open a possibility for explanation of the mechanism of PR potentiation in atria. Ca^{2+} released during rest from mitochondria may be taken up by the SR and subsequently released at the first PR excitation augmenting greatly the CF. Following this it is extruded from the cell, which results in emptying of both those compartments and brings about a sudden decline of CF of the next beats. The last statement concerning Ca^{2+} extrusion has been strongly supported by experiments based on different methods (Bers & MacLeod, 1986; Hilgemann, 1986a, 1986b). Some additional experimental evidence will be needed to evaluate the hypothesis presented above concerning the origin of calcium related to PR potentiation in atria, whether mitochondria might be, at least partly, a possible cellular site of Ca_2 fraction, which primes the potentiated PRC.

References

Bers, D.M. (1983). Early transient depletion of extracellular Ca during individual cardiac muscle contractions. *Am. J. Physiol.*, **244**, H462-H468.

Bers, D.M. (1985). Ca influx and sarcoplasmic reticulum Ca release in cardiac muscle activation during postrest recovery. *Am. J. Physiol.*, **248**, H366-H381.

Bers, D.M, & MacLeod, K.T. (1986). Cumulative depletions of extracellular calcium in rabbit ventricular muscle monitored with calcium sensitive microelectrodes. *Circ. Res.*, **58**, 769-782.

Capogrossi, M.C., Kort, A.A., Spurgeon, H.A., & Lakatta, E.G. (1986). Single adult rabbit and rat cardiac myocytes retain the Ca- and species-dependent systolic and diastolic contractile properties of intact muscle. *J. Gen. Physiol.*, **88**, 589-613.

Chapman, R.A. (1983). Control of cardiac contractility at the cellular level. *Am. J. Physiol.*, **245**, H535-H552.

Chapman, R.A., & Niedergerke, R. (1970). Interaction between heart rate and calcium concentration in the control of contractile strength of the frog heart. *J. Physiol. Lond.*, **211**, 423-443.

Hilgemann, D.W. (1986a). Extracellular calcium transients and action potential configuration changes related to post-stimulatory potentiation in rabbit atrium. *J. Gen. Physiol.*, **87**, 675-706.

Hilgemann, D.W. (1986b). Extracellular calcium transients at single excitations in rabbit atrium measured with tetramethylmurexide. *J. Gen. Physiol.*, **87**, 707-735.

Janczewski, A.M., & Lewartowski, B. (1986). The effect of prolonged rest on calcium exchange and contractions in rat and guinea-pig ventricular myocardium. *J. Mol. Cel. Cardiol.*, **18**, 1233-1242.

Koch-Weser, J., & Blinks, J.R. (1963). The influence of the interval between beats on mammalian contractility. *Pharmacological Rev.*, **15**, 601-652.

Langer, G.A. (1965). Calcium exchange in dog ventricular muscle: Relation to frequency of contraction and maintenance of contractility. *Circ. Res.*, **17**, 78-89.

Langer, G.A., & Nudd, L.M. (1980). Addition and kinetic characterization of mitochondrial calcium in myocardial tissue culture. *Am. J. Physiol.*, **239**, H769-H774.

Lehninger, A.L., Vercesi, A., & Bababuni, E.A. (1978). Regulation of Ca^{2+} release from mitochondria by the oxidation-reduction state of pyridine nucleotides. *Proc. Natl. Acad. Sci. USA*, **75**, 1690-1694.

Lewartowski, B., Pytkowski, B., & Janczewski, A.M. (1984). Calcium fraction correlating with contractile force of ventricular muscle of guinea-pig heart. *Pflügers Arch.*, **401**, 198-203.

Manning, A., & Hollander, P.B. (1971). The interval-strength relationship in mammalian atrium: A calcium exchange model. *Biophys. J.*, **11**, 483-501.

Prokopczuk, A. (1986). Localization of contractile calcium in guinea-pig atria, abstract. *J. Mol. Cell. Cardiol.*, **18**(Suppl. 3), 58.

Prokopczuk, A. (1987). Calcium shifts accompanying rest-dependent phenomena in atrial muscle of guinea-pig heart. *Acta Physiol. Pol.*, **38**, 506-515.

Prokopczuk, A., & Lewartowski, B. (1985). The effects of acetylcholine and catecholamines on post-rest phenomena in rabbit and guinea-pig atria and on accompanying shifts of ^{45}Ca in guinea-pig atrial muscle. *Acta Physiol. Pol.*, **36**, 138-149.

Pytkowski, B., Lewartowski, B., Prokopczuk, A., Zdanowski, K., & Lewandowska, K. (1983). Excitation- and rest-dependent shifts of Ca in guinea-pig ventricular myocardium. *Pflügers Arch.*, **398**, 103-113.

Rasmussen, C.A.F. Jr., Sutko, J.L., & Barry, W.H. (1987). Effects of ryanodine and caffeine on contractility, membrane voltage, and calcium exchange in cultured heart cells. *Circ. Res.*, **60**, 495-504.

Simurda, J., Simurdova, M., Braveny, P., & Sumbera, J. (1981). Activity-dependent changes of slow inward current in ventricular heart muscle. *Pflügers Arch.*, **391**, 277-283.

Takashima, K.H., Shinizu, H., Setaka, M., & Kwan, T. (1980). A spin-label study of the effects of drugs on calcium release from isolated sarcoplasmic reticulum vesicles. *J. Biochem.*, **87**, 305-312.

Weber, A., & Herz, R. (1968). The relationship between caffeine contracture of intact muscle and the effect of caffeine on reticulum. *J. Gen. Physiol.*, **52**, 750-759.

RESEARCH NOTES

The Influence of Partial Sensory Neural Blockade on Cardiovascular and Ventilatory Responses in Exercising Humans

M. Kjaer, N.H. Secher, A. Fernandes, S. Thomas, H. Galbo, and J.H. Mitchell

Department of Medical Physiology B and Department of Anaesthesia Ragshospitalet, University of Copenhagen, Denmark and Harry S. Moss Heart Center, Departments of Internal Medicine and Physiology, University of Texas, Health Science Center, Dallas

During exercise the cardiovascular and respiratory responses increase with the intensity of physical activity, and experiments have indicated that both central neural mechanisms ("central command", feed-forward control) and reflex neural mechanisms (peripheral feedback) are involved in the regulation of these responses (Asmussen et al., 1965; Eldridge et al., 1985; Mitchell, 1985).

We investigated the role of afferent nervous feedback from working muscles during dynamic exercise in humans. Small doses of epidural anaesthesia were given in order to block the thin sensoric afferent nerve fibers, leaving the thicker efferent fibers and, subsequently, motoric function almost intact.

Material and Methods

Six healthy males (30, 20-42 yrs; 80, 65-95 kg, and 179, 173-186 cm; mean and range) performed submaximal exercise (58% $\dot{V}O_2$max) for 20 min on a modified bicycle ergometer without (Co) as well as, on a separate day, during lumbar epidural anaesthesia (Ep). After the 20-min period both in Co and in Ep experiments subjects rested for 10 min before they performed graded bicycle exercise to exhaustion, work load being increased every 2 min by 50 W. To induce epidural anaesthesia, 24 ml 0.25% bupivacaine was injected to the epidural space between vertebrae L_3 and L_4. This resulted in (a) a sensoric blockade to the level of vertebrae Th 11-12 determined by pin prick, (b) an attenuation of the post-exercise ischemic pressor response (from 37 to 16 mmHg), (c) a maintenance of muscle strength on 80 $\pm$ 5% (mean and SE) of control value, and (d) no change in resting values of heart rate or mean arterial blood pressure. Intensity of effort during exercise was quantified by rating of perceived exertion on the Borg scale, blood pressure was measured in a radial artery, and plasma catecholamine concentrations were determined in arterialized blood drawn from a heated hand vein. Wilcoxon ranking test for paired data was used for statistical analysis.

Results

During submaximal exercise, rate of perceived exertion was slightly increased in Ep compared to Co experiments. Ventilation and heart rate responses were similar in Ep and Co experiments, whereas mean arterial blood pressure response was reduced during sensory nerve blockade. Results obtained in one subject indicated that sensory blockade reduced plasma norepinephrine and epinephrine responses to submaximal exercise. During maximal exercise and maximal rates of perceived exertion, identical maximal oxygen uptake was achieved with and without sensory blockade (Table 1), and both ventilation and heart rate responses were identical in Ep and Co experiments. However, blood pressure response was markedly reduced in Ep compared to Co experiments. Catecholamine responses, measured in one subject were not reduced by epidural anaesthesia.

Table 1 Cardiovascular and Respiratory Responses to Maximal Dynamic Exercise

	Control		Sensory blockade	
	Rest	Max. exercise	Rest	Max. exercise
Oxygen uptake (L • min⁻¹)		3.25 ± 0.32		3.13 ± 0.40
Ventilation (L • min⁻¹)		128 ± 13		116 ± 11
Heart rate (beats • min⁻¹)	71 ± 7	179 ± 2	69 ± 5	177 ± 1
Blood pressure (mmHg)	94 ± 5	159 ± 13	93 ± 6	$133 \pm 10*$

Note. Values are means $\pm$ *SE*. 6 subjects bicycled to exhaustion with (9.0 $\pm$ 0.8 min) as well as without epidural anaesthesia (10.8 $\pm$ 0.5 min).
*denotes difference ($p < .05$) between epidural and control experiments.

Discussion

It has earlier been found that blockade of fine afferent fibers from exercising muscle causes an abolition of the postexercise ischaemic pressor response (Freund et al., 1979), and we used this criterion to indicate a successful sensory blockade. During submaximal exercise blood pressure response was reduced when sensory input was impaired. Not even during maximal exercise could central factors compensate for the lack of sensory input (Table 1). This was probably not due to blockade of efferent sympathetic nerves to the legs since maximal norepinephrine levels measured in one subject were not reduced during epidural anaesthesia. In experiments using partial neuromuscular blockade, which weakens skeletal muscle and probably increases motor center activity necessary to produce a certain work output, the role of the central factors in blood pressure control during exercise has been evaluated. These experiments have shown that although central factors play some role in blood pressure regulation during static exercise (Leonard et al., 1985), the peripheral factors rather than motor center activity are controlling blood pressure response during dynamic exercise (Galbo et al., 1987; Kjaer et al., 1987). This agrees with the observation that although an enhanced central command during dynamic exercise is found during epidural anaesthesia compared to control exercise, it does not compensate for a lack of input from fine muscle afferents (Table 1). The fact that catecholamines do not precisely correlate with pressor responses suggests that cardiovascular dynamics during exercise are influenced by other factors than catecholamines (Kjaer et al., 1987). Ventilatory and heart rate responses to dynamic exercise were not altered by epidural anaesthesia, indicating that afferent impulses from working muscles are not crucial for these responses.

It has been shown in animal experiments (Eldridge et al., 1985) and in human studies using neuromuscular blockade (Asmussen et al., 1965; Kjaer et al., 1987) that central command plays a role in regulation of ventilation during dynamic exercise. Thus, in experiments with epidural anaesthesia, reduced peripheral input to ventilatory centers during exercise may be compensated for by increased central command. Ambiguous evidence exists as to the role of central command in the heart response to dynamic exercise (Eldridge et al., 1985; Galbo et al., 1987; Kjaer et al., 1987). One explanation for the finding of similar heart rate responses during exercise in experiments with and without the sensory blockade is that the effect of the blockade was compensated for by a decrease in the baroreceptor inhibition of heart rate due to the reduced blood pressure response in Ep as compared to Co experiments. From this study it is concluded that during dynamic exercise a normal blood pressure response is dependent on an intact sensory input.

Acknowledgments

This study was supported by the Danish Heart Foundation, Danish Medical Research Council, University of Dallas, Texas, The NOVO Foundation, Lanson and Regas Lacy Research Foundation in Cardiovascular Diseases, LaCours Foundation, and the P. Carl Petersen Foundation. We thank Lisbeth Kall for the excellent technical assistance.

References

Asmussen, E., Johansen, S.H., Jørgensen, M., & Nielsen, M. (1965). On the nervous factors controlling respiration and circulation during exercise: Experiments with curarization. *Acta Physiol. Scand.*, **63**, 343-350.

Eldrige, F.L., Milhron, E.E., Kiley, J.P., & Waldrop, G. (1985). Stimulation by central command of locomotion, respiration and circulation during exercise. *Resp. Physiol.*, **59**, 313-337.

Freund, P.M., Rowell, L.B., Murphy, T.M., Hobbs, S.F., & Butler, S.H. (1979). Blockade of the pressor response to muscle ischemia by sensory nerve block in man. *Am. J. Physiol.*, **236**, H433-H439.

Galbo, H., Kjaer, M., & Secher, N.H. (1987). Cardiovascular, ventilatory and catecholamine responses to maximal dynamic exercise in partially curarized man. *J. Physiol. (London)*, **389**, 557-568.

Kjaer, M., Secher, N.H., Bach, F.W., & Galbo, H. (1987). Role of motor center activity for hormonal changes and substrate mobilization in exercising man. *Am. J. Physiol.*, **253**, R687-R695.

Leonard, B., Mitchell, J.H., Mizuno, M., Rube, N., Saltin, B., & Secher, N.H. (1985). Partial neuromuscular blockade and cardiovascular responses to static exercise in man. *J. Physiol. (London)*, **359**, 365-379.

Mitchell, J.H. (1985). Cardiovascular control during exercise: Central and reflex neural mechanisms. *Am. J. Cardiol.*, **55**, 34D-41D.

The Relationship Between Carotid Pulse Curve and Changes in Arterial Pressure During Static Exercise

J. Siwiński, K. Kałużyński, B. Skórka, S. Kozłowski, and H. Chlebus
Institute of Internal Medicine, Medical Academy of Warsaw, Institute of Precision and Electronic Equipment Design, Technical University of Warsaw, and the Medical Research Centre, Polish Academy of Sciences, Warsaw, Poland

The analysis of carotid sphygmogram pattern was until now applied to evaluate the changes of distensibility of central arteries in the subjects with atherosclerosis and arterial hypertension (Chlebus, 1979; Chlebus et al., 1981; Valtneris, 1974). The sphygmograms, picked up with noncontact transducers, give good representation of the changes of intraarterial pressure (Summa, 1978; Taylor & Gerrard, 1977).

The value of index e in healthy subjects is always greater than 1; the angle between the upstroke part and plateau is always acute, approaching 90 degrees in cases close to pathology, and the value of index d is always smaller than 1. In patients with atherosclerosis or arterial hypertension the values of the above mentioned parameters are, respectively, smaller than 1, obtuse, and greater than 1. The reason is a decreased distensibility of central arteries. A marked decrease of the upstroke time $t1$ is found in patients in comparison with healthy subjects.

The above mentioned criteria are significantly correlated with the pulse wave velocity in the aorta. Their diagnostic value has been confirmed by the results of x-ray and anatomo-pathological examinations as well as by the experiments performed on animals (Chlebus, 1979).

The arterial wall may also be stretched because of a temporary rise in blood pressure, due to, for example, physical effort. An increase of pressure, stretching the arterial wall, decreases its distensibility, which is seen in the diminution of e value. Therefore, the index e may be considered as a measure of arterial distensibility during the examination.

The correction of index e with the relative value of mean arterial pressure enables evaluation of the arterial distensibility related to normal mean arterial pressure (Chlebus et al., 1981). The adjustment is given by the formula:

$$e_1 = e \times P_m/P_{om} \tag{1}$$

where:

e_1 = corrected index of elasticity;
P_m = mean arterial pressure during the examination;
P_{om} = average epidemiological value of mean arterial pressure of healthy subjects, arbitrarily adopted, 100 mmHg.

Supposing that e_1 is a constant value for a given state of the subject's arteries, independent of instantaneous pressure, the relationship (1) may be transformed into the following:

$$e = A/P_m \qquad (2)$$

where:

$A = e_1 \times P_{om} = $ const. for a given subject.

This relation may be used to calculate one of the values e or P_m, the second being measured, provided that the subject's constant A has been established. One of the objectives of this work was to verify the above hypothesis.

Material and Methods

The examinations were carried out on 10 healthy male volunteers, aged 22 to 33 years. The measurements were made in a supine position after 15 min of rest. In each case the carotid pulse signal was recorded using a noncontact capacitive modulation transducer. Blood pressure was simultaneously measured according to the Korotkoff method. The carotid pulse signal and pressure were measured at rest and during static handgrip exercise. Each person performed the exercise with a force equal to 30% of his MVC (maximal voluntary contraction). The time of exercise (to exhaustion) varied from 6 to 10 minutes.

The measurements of blood pressure and the carotid pulse signal recordings were carried out every 90 seconds. The carotid sphygmogram was recorded on a recorder with bandwidth from DC to 800 Hz. The registered signal served to calculate the indices of elasticity and of the mean arterial pressure (by integration of the area below the carotid pulse curve calibrated with systolic and diastolic pressure). Those parameters were averaged from five consecutive cardiac cycles. Each value of e was corrected according to the current mean arterial pressure, providing the value of corresponding index e_1. The maximum increase of mean arterial pressure and the corresponding change of e value were calculated in each case. The correlation coefficient r between the e and P was calculated and the relation (2) was evaluated for each subject.

Results

The application of static exercise met both the physiological and technical requirements. Such exercise, especially when the upper extremities are involved, gives a fast and large increase of mean arterial pressure (Brorson et al., 1979; Helfant et al., 1971; Lind, 1970).

The results of calculations and statistical analysis are presented in Table 1. The dynamics of pulse curve changes Δe is significant in all cases. The increase in mean arterial pressure ΔP_m is significant in all subjects and reaches 55% of its initial value. The values of the elasticity index e exceeded 1 at the beginning of the exercise in all but two subjects, where values were only slightly smaller than 1. Thus, the proper choice of subjects has been confirmed. The decrease of e value follows the mean pressure increase in all cases. The decrease of elasticity index e corresponds to the increase of the mean arterial pressure. The correlation coefficient r between the values of e and P_m is below 0.90 in all but two subjects. The quotient of standard deviation to mean value of $e_1[SD/m(e_1)]$ does not exceed 9% in any instant of the experiment in spite of the changes of mean arterial pressure.

Table 1 Results of Examinations and Analysis

No.	Subject, age	P_m (mmHg) Initial	P_m (mmHg) Final	e Initial	e Final	ΔP_m	Δe	r	e_1	$SD/m(e_1)$	Relationship between a and P_m
1	KG, 25	98	127	1.80	1.21	29	−0.59	−0.92	1.55 ± 0.110	0.0708	e = 162/P
2	WT, 26	117	135	0.98	0.62	18	−0.36	−0.86	1.05 ± 0.040	0.0387	e = 103/P
3	AL, 22	100	148	1.12	0.85	48	−0.27	−0.95	1.21 ± 0.068	0.0565	e = 120/P
4	JW, 24	98	126	1.44	1.13	28	−0.31	−0.99	1.42 ± 0.017	0.0133	e = 142/P
5	SS, 23	100	130	1.30	0.93	30	−0.37	−0.95	1.29 ± 0.065	0.0504	e = 130/P
6	KK, 30	91	123	0.97	0.64	32	−0.33	−0.99	0.82 ± 0.069	0.0841	e = 83/P
7	GF, 23	103	130	1.50	1.00	27	−0.50	−0.98	1.35 ± 0.055	0.0408	e = 138/P
8	LS, 33	118	142	1.21	0.85	24	−0.36	−0.92	1.40 ± 0.035	0.0252	e = 139/P
9	MK, 27	97	149	1.26	0.91	52	−0.35	−0.78	1.34 ± 0.060	0.0450	e = 136/P
10	EK, 31	103	130	1.25	1.02	27	−0.23	−0.99	1.33 ± 0.040	0.0300	e = 133/P

The individual hyperbolic relationships between the index e and the mean arterial pressure for each subject are given in Table 1. The results of measurements in 2 subjects and the corresponding hyperbolic functions confirm the good accuracy of proposed relationship between the index e and the mean arterial pressure.

Discussion

The changes of carotid pulse pattern observed during the static exercise are caused by the increase of the mean arterial pressure and are in accordance with previously reported properties of the arterial wall (Busse et al., 1979; McDonald, 1974; O'Rourke, 1982; Taylor & Gerrard, 1977). The changes of carotid pulse pattern result from an increase of the value of the Young modulus, the latter caused by the elevated arterial pressure. Those changes have an individual character. The index e, decreasing with an increase of the mean arterial pressure, describes the compliance (distensibility) of the arterial wall and yields a quantitative measure of those changes. The carotid pulse patterns found in all subjects at the end of the static exercise, when the mean arterial pressure was substantially increased, are abnormal, as they would be in the case of atherosclerosis.

The index e_1 has a physical meaning of compliance for normal mean arterial pressure. Therefore, one may expect it to be a constant value, characteristic for a given subject. This has been proved by the results of the examinations. The standard deviation of e_1 does not exceed 9% of its mean value in any case. The spread of e_1 values may be due, in major part, to the measurement inaccuracies, for example, of the Korotkoff method. Thus, the index e_1 may be considered as a constant value relating the mean arterial pressure to the index e, describing current carotid pulse pattern and distensibility. The product of e_1, once calculated according to formula (1), and of the normal mean arterial pressure may be used to evaluate the actual mean arterial pressure on the basis of carotid pulse curve, or, inversely, to estimate the instantaneous compliance of the arterial wall on the basis of mean arterial pressure, according to formula (2).

However, the constant character of the index e_1 may be assumed in time periods sufficiently short to neglect the effects of physiological aging (O'Rourke, 1982). The possibility of evaluating the mean arterial pressure on the basis of carotid pulse pattern and vice versa may be of great importance in clinical practice and research.

Conclusions

1. The increase of mean arterial pressure causes a change of carotid pulse pattern, seen as a diminution of the value of index e.

2. The index e_1, which is insensitive to the changes of the mean arterial pressure, allows one to estimate the compliance of the arterial wall related to the anatomical state of the vessel, independently of the variations of blood pressure during the examination.

3. The index e_1 may be considered as a constant value for a given subject, which describes quantitatively the relationship between the carotid pulse pattern and the mean arterial pressure.

References

Brorson, L., Wasir, H., & Sannerstedt, R. (1979). Haemodynamic effects of static and dynamic exercise in males with arterial hypertension of varying severity. *Cardiovasc. Res.*, **12**, 269-275.

Busse, R., Bauer, R.D., Schabert, A., Summa, Y., Bumm, P., & Wetterer, E. (1979). The mechanical properties of exposed human common carotid arteries "in vivo." *Basic Research in Cardiology*, **74**, 545-554.

Chlebus, H. (1979). Clinical application of carotid electrosphygmography. *Biblthca. Cardiol.*, **37**, 73-83.

Chlebus, H., Siwiński, J., Skórka, B., & Kałużyński, K. (1981). Estimation of pattern of carotid pulse signal in comparison with blood pressure and blood flow parameters. *Biocybernetics and Biomedical Engineering*, **1**, 19-31.

Helfant, R., de Villa, M., & Meister, S. (1971). Effects of sustained isometric handgrip exercise on left ventricular performance. *Circulation*, **44**, 982-1002.

Lind, A. (1970). Cardiovascular responses to static exercise. *Circulation*, **44**, 173-176.

McDonald, D.A. (1974). Pulsative flow in an elastic tube. In E. Arnold (Ed.), *Blood flow in arteries*, 298-308.

O'Rourke, M.F. (1982). Contour of the arterial pulse and its interpretation. In *Arterial function in health and disease*, Churchill Livingstone, 132-152.

Taylor, A.L., & Gerrard, J.H. (1977). Pressure-radius relationships for elastic tubes and their application to arteries. *Part I. Med. and Biol. Eng. and Comput.*, **15**, 11-17.

Summa, Y. (1978). Determination of tangential elastic modulus of human arteries "in vivo." In R.D. Bauer & R. Busse (Eds.), *The arterial system*, Springer, 95-100.

Valtneris, A.D. (1974). Change of the sphygmogram form under the influence of physical load according to the contour analysis data. *Sechenov Physiological Journal of the USSR*, **60**, 1235-1240.

Anaerobic Performance and Arterial Blood Pressure in Healthy Men

M. Szczypaczewska

Department of Clinical and Applied Physiology, School of Medicine, Warsaw, Poland

There are data suggesting an increased incidence of hypertension among people with a high percentage of fast twitching (FT) fibers in skeletal muscles (Juhlin-Dannfelt et al., 1979); on the other hand, it is known that such muscle fiber composition plays a role in determining anaerobic performance (Bar-Or et al., 1980). Thus, the present study was designed to find out whether young, healthy subjects with high anaerobic capacity show any hemodynamic abnormalities that can be considered as pregoing symptoms of hypertension.

Material and Methods

Twenty seven strength-trained (S) subjects (body builders and weight lifters), 20 endurance trained (E) and 20 untrained (U) subjects volunteered for this study. Their main characteristics are given in Table 1, the subjects' anaerobic capacity was determined using the Wingate test.

All the subjects performed 18-min graded (3×6) bicycle-ergometer exercise with work loads of 50, 100, and 150 W. At the end of each load heart rate (HR), blood pressure (BP) and cardiac output ($\dot{Q}$—by CO_2 rebreathing method) were measured. Besides, venous blood samples were taken for determinations of the plasma catecholamines (NA and A),

Table 1 Characteristics of Subjects

Groups		Age (years)	Weight (kg)	Height (cm)	Body fat (%)	$\dot{V}O_2$max (L $\cdot$ min^{-1})	Resting BP (mmHg) Syst.	Diast.
S	$\bar{x}$	25	78.2	177	7.5	3.27	125	80
	SD	5.6	12.0	6	1.2	0.49	11	7
E	$\bar{x}$	20	66.7	175	6.8	3.77	116	74
	SD	0.7	4.5	6	0.7	0.51	6	8
U	$\bar{x}$	24	73.6	176	14.5	2.84	113	74
	SD	4	5.3	10	5.8	0.52	6	6

renin activity (PRA), vasopressin (ADH), and cortisol. Plasma catecholamines were measured radioenzymatically, whereas PRA, ADH, and cortisol used radioimmunoassays. In additional experiments HR and BP responses to the static handgrip, at 30% of maximal voluntary contraction (MVC), were examined in all three groups of subjects.

Results and Discussion

Blood pressure at rest in the strength-trained subjects was slightly, but significantly, higher in comparison with the other 2 groups (Table 1). They showed also significantly higher maximal and total power output during the Wingate test.

During submaximal dynamic exercise S-subjects reached significantly greater BP, $\dot{Q}$, and stroke volume (SV) in comparison with the remaining groups. No significant differences between groups were found in the calculated total peripheral resistance (TPR). In strength-trained subjects BP responses to static exercise were also elevated.

A significant relationship was ascertained between the subjects' anaerobic capacity/total power output during the Wingate test and BP response to dynamic (150 W) exercise. No differences between groups were demonstrated in the hormonal responses to dynamic exercise. It should be noted that the highest blood cortisol levels were found in S-group ($p < .05$).

This work demonstrated that healthy young men of high anaerobic capacity have slightly higher blood pressure at rest, and their BP response to both dynamic and static exercises is exaggerated. This can be attributed to increased cardiac output and is not associated with any appreciable alterations in the plasma catecholamine and ADH levels or the plasma renin activity.

The mechanism of the relationship between anaerobic capacity and the hemodynamic responses to exercise remains unclear. It is also unknown whether the differences in these responses between strength and endurance-trained or sedentary subjects reflect the specific training effects or the genetically determined characteristics such as muscle fiber distribution.

Since it has been proved (Wilson & Meyer, 1981) that the recognition of an elevated blood pressure response to exercise in persons with a normal BP at rest provides a means for early identification of hypertension-prone individuals, the present data suggest that high anaerobic capacity is connected in some way with a predisposition toward hypertension.

References

Bar-Or, O., Dotan, R., Inbar, O., Rothstein, A., Karlsson, J., & Tesch, P. (1980). Anaerobic capacity and muscle fiber distribution in man. *Int. J. Sport Med.*, **1**, 82-85.

Juhlin-Dannfelt, A., Frisk-Holmberg, M., Karlsson, J., & Tesch, P. (1979). Central and peripheral circulation in relation to muscle-fibre composition in normo- and hypertensive man. *Clin. Sci.*, **56**, 335-340.

Wilson, N.V., & Meyer, B.M. (1981). Early prediction of hypertension using exercise blood pressure. *Preventive Med.*, **10**, 62-68.

Exercise Adaptation of the Circulatory System Under Low-Oxygen Mixture Breathing

K. Mazurek, R. Dabrowa, A. Orzel, and J. Piórko

Military Institute of Aviation Medicine, Warsaw, Poland

The evaluation of a pilot's aptitude for aviation is based, among other criteria, on examining adaptation of his circulatory system to different environmental stressors. In selected cases exercise tests with low-oxygen mixture breathing are applied. In the present study, 12% oxygen–nitrogen mixture was used, during a 15-min ergometer exercise test. The exercise load was linearly increasing by 0.7 W per second, up to the heart rate (HR) of 160 • min^{-1}. The assigned level of the "steady state" HR was maintained using the biofeedback technique (HR-load). In the evaluation of exercise adaptation, the following variables were included: HR, systolic and diastolic arterial blood pressure (BP$_s$, BP$_d$), peripheral resistance (R), and physical load (W). In the postexercise restitution period, additional polycardiographic indices were measured. The data were analyzed for two extremal groups of pilots, representing different levels of performance capacity.

It was found that breathing the hypoxic mixture at rest produces a moderate rise in HR, a slight decrease of the peripheral vascular resistance, and a small decrease of stroke volume without any significant changes in the cardiac index. Similarly, decreases of the QS$_2$I, LVETI, PEP, and ICT values without changes in the contractility index PEP/LVET were observed.

During exercise under hypoxic conditions work tolerance of the examined pilots was reduced as evidenced by a decrease in the maximal power of the performed work (W$_{max160}$) by 13% and in the total work performed (W$_{15}$). The maximal power of work and the total work performed may be regarded, similar to maximum oxygen uptake (V̇O$_2$max), as indicators of exercise tolerance. Comparing the exercise tolerance in pilots of high (group A) and low (group B) fitness, it was found that during 15 min of exercise in hypoxia, pilots from group A performed 22% more work at the same HR (160 • min^{-1}) than pilots from group B. In hypoxia the time of achieving the assigned-in-advance HR (t$_{max}$HR) was evidently prolonged with lower value of W$_{max160}$. Well, fit pilots achieved HR 160 • min^{-1} after a longer time. This suggests better adaptation ability of the cardiovascular system in those subjects (Åstrand, 1976).

Adaptation of the cardiovascular system to exercise was characterized, moreover, by lower values of diastolic arterial blood pressure and peripheral resistance. These results agree with those reported by other authors (Bujanow & Pisarienko, 1975).

The stroke volume after exercise in hypoxia was larger than in the control test while the trend of its changes was similar (Goldberg & Shephard, 1980). In the group of pilots of low physical fitness, an increased stroke volume was found 30 seconds and 3 minutes after exercise under hypoxic conditions, and the absolute values of this variable were always lower than in the well, fit subjects.

Comparing the polycardiographic parameters at the time of postexercise restitution with their resting values, a decrease in the values of PEP, ICT, and PEP/LVET index was observed from the 30th second to the 3rd minute after exercise. These parameters achieved values approaching the normal ones after 5 to 10 minutes. Changes of the left-ventricular contraction periods found immediately after the exercise performed in hypoxia have been termed the "hyperdynamic syndrome." The complex of changes found in this study in the subjects of low physical fitness, in the late restitution period (35th minute), has been termed "the phase of hypodynamia" (Cholewa, 1978).

Conclusions

1. Hypoxia modifies exercise tolerance, decreasing power and the total work performed at the assigned HR.

2. Adaptation of the cardiovascular system to exercise under hypoxic conditions is characterized by earlier achievement of the assigned HR, lower diastolic arterial pressure, and decreased peripheral resistance.

3. The observed differences in the response of the cardiovascular system to exercise in hypoxia depend on the subjects' physical fitness. Well, fit pilots performed more work at a given HR and showed greater exercise tolerance in hypoxia.

4. Highly fit subjects showed more pronounced hyperdynamic response immediately after exercise while in those of low fitness, a hypodynamic response appeared later on during the restitution.

References

Åstrand, P.O. (1976). Quantification of exercise capability and evaluation of physical capacity in man. *Progress in Cardiovascular Disease, 19,* 51.

Bujanow, P.W., & Pisarienko, N.W. (1975). Evaluation of physical work load tests on basis of hemodynamic indices. *Journal of Military Medicine* (in Russian), **12,** 69.

Cholewa, M. (1978). *Combined cardiometric and biochemical studies during recovery from physical exercise: Effects of some drugs.* Central Military-Medical Library, Military School of Medicine, Łódź (in Polish).

Goldberg, D.I., & Shephard, R.I. (1980). Stroke volume during recovery from upright bicycle exercise. *Journal of Applied Physiology,* **48,** 833.

Adaptation of Cardiovascular Function in the Course of Endurance Training of Moderate Intensity in Healthy Men

K. Krzemiński and K. Nazar

Department of Applied Physiology, Medical Research Centre, Polish Academy of Sciences, Warsaw, Poland

Eighteen male volunteers (20-23 years) were submitted to 13-week training consisting of 30 min exercise at 50 to 75% $\dot{V}O_2$max on a bicycle ergometer performed three times a week. Every 3 to 4 weeks cardiac function was evaluated by left ventricle systolic time interval measurements at rest, during submaximal bicycle exercises, and static handgrip. Besides, $\dot{V}O_2$max, anaerobic threshold (AT), maximal stroke volume (SV_{max}), and blood pressure (BP) responses to dynamic and static exercises were determined. Significant increases in $\dot{V}O_2$max, AT, and SV_{max} as well as decreases in submaximal heart rate (HR) and BP responses to static and dynamic exercises were found already after 4 weeks of training. Resting systolic time intervals were not affected by training. However, during dynamic and static exercise the preejection period and isovolumic contraction time interval were significantly shortened after 8 weeks of training, when compared at the same HR. It is concluded that endurance training of moderate intensity improves cardiac function during dynamic exercise performed with trained muscles and during static exercise performed with untrained muscles.

Cardiovascular and Sympatho-Adrenal Responses to Static Handgrip Performed With One and Two Hands

R. Grucza, G. Cybulski, J.F. Kahn, W. Niewiadomski,
E. Stupnicka, and K. Nazar

Department of Applied Physiology, Medical Research Centre, Polish Academy of Sciences, Warsaw, Poland and Laboratoire de Physiologie du Tavail, CNRS, Paris, France

The study was performed to follow up the changes in stroke volume (SV) measured by impedance reography in healthy men during static exercise and to evaluate the relationships between the muscle mass involved in the effort, magnitude of cardiovascular response, and changes in plasma catecholamine concentrations. Twelve healthy male subjects aged 21 to 25 years participated in the study. They performed static handgrip at 25 to 30% maximal voluntary contraction (MVC) with one and two hands. Both one-hand and two-hand exercise caused a marked SV reduction. There were no significant differences either in the magnitude of this response or in the changes in heart rate, blood pressure, and plasma catecholamine concentration occurring during handgrip performed with one and two hands. The study indicates, therefore, that the cardiovascular and sympatho-adrenal responses to static handgrip, at a given percentage of MVC, do not depend on the muscle mass involved in the effort.

Part II
Exercise Metabolism and Performance

Regulation of Glycogen Metabolism in Exercising Muscle

E. Hultman, J.M. Ren, and L.L. Spriet

Karolinska Institute, Huddinge University Hospital, Huddinge, Sweden

Despite ATP being the sole energy source during contraction, the level of this metabolite remains essentially constant during exercise. The obvious conclusion is that muscle, in response to the contraction, is able to raise its level of ATP production to match the rate of utilization.

The muscles have essentially four ways of producing ATP: (a) from phosphocreatine at a maximum rate of 150 mmol ATP • min^{-1} • kg^{-1} muscle, (b) from glycolysis at a maximum rate of 84 mmol ATP • min^{-1} • kg^{-1} muscle, (c) from oxidation of pyruvate at a maximum rate of 36 mmol ATP • min^{-1} • kg^{-1} muscle, and (d) from free fatty acid oxidation at a rate of 15 mmol ATP • min^{-1} • kg^{-1} muscle. The estimates of maximum utilization of fuels are given for a typical human (Hultman & Sjöholm, 1986; McGilvery, 1975). The rate of fat oxidation can be increased by endurance training. Without doubt carbohydrate is quantitatively the most important of these four fuel sources during prolonged intense muscular effort.

It would seem relatively easy today to explain in principle the mechanisms by which glycolysis is coordinated with the rate of ATP utilization—with control being exercised at the level of phosphofructokinase (PFK) and pyruvate dehydrogenase (PDH). However, this presentation will try to focus on a more difficult and contentious problem; namely, the regulation of glycogenolysis itself, which of course provides the basic units of glycolysis.

Glycogenolysis During Exercise

With the start of exercise, glycogen phosphorylase is activated and in the presence of inorganic phosphate glycogen is broken down to hexose-P. Despite the simultaneous activation of PFK, the initial rate of glycogenolysis is always higher than the glycolytic rate resulting in the accumulation of hexose-P. During prolonged submaximal exercise, however, the glycogenolytic rate decreases continuously to rates equal to or even lower than the rate of glycolysis. This is observed as a discontinuation of the initial hexose-P increase with successively decreasing concentrations during continued exercise (Hultman & Bergström, 1973; Hultman & Spriet, 1986).

It is well known that the glycogenolytic rate during dynamic exercise is directly related to the work load. Figure 1 shows the glycogenolytic rates in a series of studies in which dynamic exercise was performed to exhaustion with loads that could be sustained for periods of 30 seconds to 1 hour. Glycogenolytic rates ranged from 40 mmol • min^{-1} • kg^{-1} to 1.4 mmol • min^{-1} • kg^{-1}. The maximum rate observed, 40 mmol • min^{-1} • kg^{-1} is close to the $\dot{V}_{max}$ of the phosphorylase enzyme as determined in human quadriceps muscle (Chasiotis, 1983). The variation in rate is related to the work intensity and can be explained by different frequencies of neural stimulation of the muscle and/or by variation of the numbers of motor units simultaneously recruited. The glycogenolytic rates in Figure 1 were calculated as mean values for the whole work periods.

Mean glycogenolytic rate,
mmol· kg⁻¹·min⁻¹

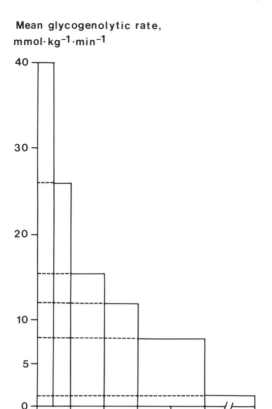

Work time, min

Figure 1. Glycogenolytic rates during maximal dynamic exercise with durations from 30 seconds to 60 min. Work loads were chosen to produce exhaustion within the predetermined times. References are listed in the same order as the different work times: Åstrand et al., 1986; Bergström et al., 1967; Boobis et al., 1982; Gollnick et al., 1973; Harris et al., 1971; Hermansen & Vaage, 1977.

When, however, the changes during 60-min dynamic exercise were analyzed in detail, it was found that the glycogenolytic rate decreased successively with time during the exercise in spite of constant work intensity. The 60-min work was divided into four 15-min periods, interrupted by biopsy sampling and separated by 15 min of rest. The glycogen degradation rates during the four work periods were 2.7, 1.4, 0.9, and 0.5 mmol • min⁻¹ • kg⁻¹ muscle. The work load was 75% of $\dot{V}O_2$max, and the whole glycogen store was utilized during the exercise (Bergström & Hultman, 1967).

It is possible to explain the low glycogenolytic rate during the final period of exercise on the basis of a lack of substrate, but not so during the earlier three periods. In these periods the mechanism could be an inhibition of the glycogenolytic process or a change in the pattern of fiber recruitment from predominantly glycolytic to more oxidative fibers.

In order to avoid the variation in stimulation frequency and the recruitment of different motor units, inherent in voluntary muscle contraction, we have used electrical stimulation of the quadriceps muscle. By this method the stimulation frequency as well as the muscle fiber population recruited is kept constant throughout the experiment. The initial glycogenolytic rate is related to the stimulation frequency with a maximum rate of approximately 40 mmol • min^{-1} • kg^{-1} at 50 Hz stimulation, similar to the rate observed during maximal dynamic exercise. At 20 Hz stimulation the initial rate is of the order of 20 to 30 mmol • min^{-1} • kg^{-1} (Hultman, 1986; Hultman & Sjöholm, 1983a, 1983b). If the stimulation, however, is prolonged the glycogenolytic rate falls rapidly. Thus, as shown by Hultman and Spriet (1986), a period of intermittent stimulation at 20 Hz for 45 min resulted in a glycogenolytic rate of 9.4 mmol • min^{-1} • kg^{-1} during the initial 1.5 min, decreasing to 1.3 mmol in the following 15 min and to 0.4 mmol • min^{-1} in the period of 15 to 45 min. During the 45 min of stimulation only 50% of the muscle glycogen store was utilized.

Regulation of Phosphorylase Activity

The glycogenolytic rate is regulated by the activity of the phosphorylase enzyme which exists in two interconvertible forms—phosphorylase b and phosphorylase a. The b form is inactive in muscle cells with a normal content of ATP and glucose-6-P but can be activated by AMP. It is generally considered that the a form of the enzyme is the only active form and determines the glycogenolytic rate both in resting and exercising muscle. The transformation of phosphorylase from b to a is mediated by a phosphorylase kinase b which is activated by Ca^{2+} increase when troponin is present. Half maximum activity of the kinase b is reached at a Ca^{2+} content of 4 μmol • L^{-1} (Cohen, 1980, 1981) which is attained in contracting muscle, while the Ca^{2+} content in resting muscle is only 0.1 μmol • L^{-1} (Perry, 1974). The phosphorylase kinase b can be transformed to kinase a via phosphorylation mediated by cyclic AMP dependent protein kinase. Phosphorylase kinase a is active at the Ca^{2+} content prevailing in resting muscle. Phosphorylase a is retransformed to b by protein phosphatase, the activity of which is regulated by a heat-stable inhibitor. The inhibitor is active only when phosphorylated, and this is mediated via cyclic AMP dependent protein kinase (Huang & Glinsmann, 1976).

The effect of a hormone-induced increase of cyclic AMP in the muscle cells is to increase the sensitivity of the phosphorylase transformation system to Ca^{2+} and simultaneously to inhibit retransformation of the a form. The enzymes involved in glycogen degradation are bound to the glycogen molecule forming a protein glycogen complex, which is also in close contact with the sarcoplasmic reticulum (Meyer et al., 1970). This provides a very tight link between Ca^{2+} and phosphorylase activation.

Phosphorylase Activity During Exercise

Upon initiation of contraction there is an immediate transformation of phosphorylase to the a form by activation of the kinase b via Ca^{2+} increase. Within the first 5 seconds of a 20-Hz intermittent stimulation the phosphorylase a fraction is increased to 70%, and after 10 to 20 seconds 90% is converted to a form. When contraction is continued, however, phosphorylase a is converted back to b, and after 3 min of contraction the fraction in the a form is once again close to the basal level. Similar results have been described for rat muscle during electrical stimulation (Conlee et al., 1979). In our own studies in humans the decline in phosphorylase a was paralleled by a fall in force output (Figure 2) and could thus be explained at least partially by a decrease in Ca^{2+} release caused by a progressive impairment of excitation-contraction coupling. In contrast, in the model of Conlee et al. (1979) using rat soleus muscle, force remained constant throughout the stimulation period. This is similar to the situation in dynamic exercise in which work output was found to be unchanged despite the fall in glycogenolytic rate. In these two cases Ca^{2+} release is probably unchanged and the results point to a dissociation between the activation of

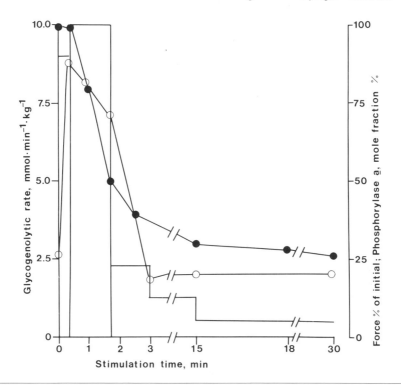

Figure 2. Glycogenolytic rate (//), phosphorylase *a* fraction (o), and force (•) during 30-min intermittent electrical stimulation at Hz.

phosphorylase and contraction. Thus, during prolonged exercise during which a physiological steady state is attained, glycogenolysis is turned down after a brief initial period and other substrates take over the muscles' energy needs (Conlee et al., 1979).

Uncoupling of Phosphorylase Activation With Contraction

One possible mechanism that could explain the uncoupling effect of exercise was suggested by Entman et al. (1980). They showed that degradation of glycogen in the glycogen-protein-sarcoplasmic reticulum complex released phosphorylase from the complex. As a result rapid glycogenolysis leads to a progressive uncoupling of phosphorylase *b* from the Ca^{2+} activation mechanism. In this model it was also suggested that the phosphorylase phosphatase was released from the glycogen complex and activated, and thus was responsible for the reversal of phosphorylase *a*. This mechanism for phosphorylase reversal was studied by Constable et al. (1986) in rat muscle using an electrical stimulation test before and after exhausting exercise. They found that partial degradation of glycogen reversed the activation of phosphorylase, but their results also pointed to a second mechanism being involved in the inhibition of phosphorylase activation. In the intermittent electrical stimulation study shown in Figure 2, reversal of the phosphorylase *a* fraction back to the basal level occurred within 3 min and remained at that level during further stimulation. Even still, glycogen degradation continued with a rate of 1.3 mmol • min^{-1} • kg^{-1} during the following 12 min. This is probably explained by the increase in inorganic phosphate (P_i), due to degradation of PCr. The P_i content in resting muscle is in the order of 2 to 3 mmol • L^{-1} cell water (Chasiotis, 1983) and the increase after a 3-min contraction was 19 mmol • L^{-1}. The K_m for P_i for phosphorylase a is 28 mmol • L^{-1} without AMP and 6.8 mmol • L^{-1} with 2 mmol AMP • L^{-1} (Chasiotis, 1983). Increase in P_i during stimulation will thus increase the activity of the phosphorylase a fraction.

Phosphorylase Activity and Adrenaline

It was shown by Chasiotis et al. (1983) that adrenaline infusion (0.14 μg • min^{-1} • kg^{-1} b.w.) increased the phosphorylase a fraction to 80 to 90% in resting muscle. If, however, the same infusion was preceded by a 60-second isometric contraction, the phosphorylase a fraction increased to only 43%. This was attributed to the fall in pH after the isometric exercise due to the lactate accumulation. The pH decrease was suggested to inhibit phosphorylase kinase (Chasiotis & Hultman, 1985; Krebs et al., 1964). However, similar blunting of the adrenaline effect was shown by Constable et al. (1986) in rat muscle taken after exhaustive dynamic exercise and persisting during more than 25 min of recovery when the pH was normalized.

In a recent study with intermittent electrical stimulation, adrenaline was infused after 15 min of stimulation (Spriet et al., 1987). The phosphorylase a fraction increased from 20 to 47% during the initial 3 min of adrenaline infusion and remained at 43% while stimulation and infusion were continued for a further 15 min. The combined effects of adrenaline infusion and Ca^{2+} were thus a lower formation of phosphorylase a than induced by adrenaline alone when given at rest (Figure 3).

The lactate content in the stimulated muscle was only 4.1 mmol • L^{-1} which excludes a fall in muscle pH alone as an explanation for the decreased response to adrenaline. There was an increase in glycogenolytic rate from 0.4 mmol • min^{-1} • kg^{-1} without adrenaline to 1.3 mmol during the infusion. The increase is, however, lower than expected from the phosphorylase fraction and the P_i content in the muscle. This suggests that both the phosphorylase transformation and the expression of the enzyme are partially inhibited in the contracting muscle—an effect of the prolonged stimulation as such or related to dissociation of the glycogen-protein complex by the initial degradation of glycogen branches.

Total Glycogen Utilization

It is well known that dynamic exercise with submaximal work loads can utilize the whole glycogen store in the muscle (Bergström & Hultman, 1967), even when this has been increased by previous exercise combined with carbohydrate loading (Bergström et al., 1967). A prolonged electrical stimulation (45 min) at 20 Hz utilized only 50% of the glycogen store, and the glycogen degradation rate was much lower in the period 15 to 45 min than during the same time period in dynamic exercise. The reason for this could be that dynamic exercise utilized alternating motor units during contraction while the same fiber population is constantly contracting during electrical stimulation. When, however, adrenaline was infused in the period 15 to 30 min of electrical stimulation, the rate of glycogenolysis increased to approximately the same rate as during the same period of the 60-min dynamic work. Increased concentration of adrenaline in blood is a regular finding, and this could at least partially explain the difference in glycogenolytic rate between dynamic exercise and electrical stimulation. Similar findings have been reported by Richter et al. (1982).

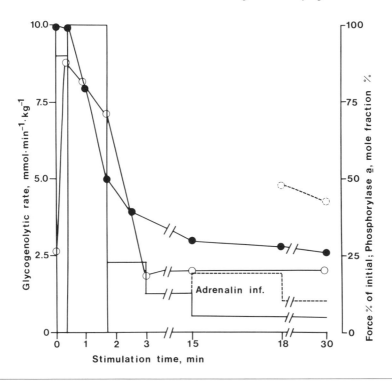

Figure 3. The same experiment and symbols as in Figure 2 but showing also the effect of adrenalin infusion during the period 15 min to 30 min (broken lines). Force generation was not changed during adrenalin infusion.

Glycogenolysis and Force Generation

As shown in Figure 3, force generation during intermittent stimulation fell rapidly to 60% of the initial within 3 min of contraction, decreased further to 30%, and remained at that level for the next 30 min. The force generation was completely unchanged during adrenaline infusion while both glycogenolytic and glycolytic rates increased with a rise in hexose-P and lactate concentration in muscle. The results indicate that the low force generation during the electrical stimulation was not due to a lack of glycolytic substrate. In a similar study (Hultman & Spriet, 1986) it was shown that initially during contraction PCr concentration decreased to 4 mmol • kg^{-1} at the 2-min contraction, but thereafter increased back to 15 mmol • kg^{-1} during continued contraction, showing that ATP production was higher than ATP utilization between 2 min and 45 min. At the same time lactate content in the working muscle decreased from 20 mmol • kg^{-1} at 2 min to 2 mmol • kg^{-1} at 45 min (see Figure 4). Apparently the low force generation cannot be attributed to lack of substrate (pyruvate or oxygen) or to lack of ATP generation during the electrical stimulation. Neither can the force decrease be attributed to changes in intramuscular milieu, such as pH decrease or accumulation of P$_i$, both suggested to be "fatigue mechanisms." The remaining cause for decreased force generation is an inhibition of excitation-contraction coupling.

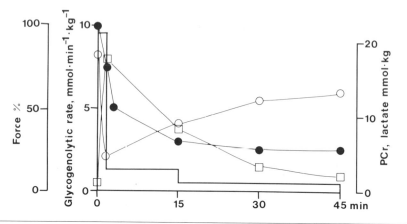

Figure 4.   Glycogenolytic rate, PCr (o), lactate concentration (□), and force generation (•) during intermittent electrical stimulation at 20 Hz. From Hultman & Spriet, 1986.

Summary

The decline in glycogenolytic rate seen during continuous exercise or prolonged electrical stimulation is due to a decreased phosphorylase *a* fraction. This is related to a fall in the Ca^{2+} stimulation of phosphorylase *b* kinase either as a result of a lower Ca^{2+} release from the sarcoplasmic reticulum or an uncoupling of the kinase-activation mechanism resulting from glycogen degradation. The decline in *a* fraction can at least partly be overcome by adrenaline infusion. The decrease in force generation observed during prolonged electrical stimulation is not due to lack of substrate for ATP production or changed intracellular milieu, but rather to inhibition of excitation-contraction coupling.

Acknowledgments

The authors wish to thank the entire staff of the Department of Clinical Chemistry II for excellent collaboration in this investigation. This work was supported by grants from the Swedish (02647) and Canadian Medical Research Councils and the Swedish Sports Research Council (44/86).

References

Åstrand, P.O., Hultman, E., Juhlin-Dannfelt, A., & Reynolds, G. (1986). Disposal of lactate during and after strenuous exercise in humans. *J. Appl. Physiol., 61*, 338-343.

Bergström, J., & Hultman, E. (1967). A study of the glycogen metabolism during exercise in man. *Scand. J. Clin. Lab. Invest., 19*, 218-228.

Bergström, J., Hermansen, L., Hultman, E., & Saltin, B. (1967). Diet, muscle glycogen and physical performance. *Acta Physiol. Scand., 71*, 140-150.

Boobis, L., Williams, C., & Wootton, S.A. (1982). Human muscle metabolism during brief maximal exercise. *J. Physiol., 338*, 21P-22P.

Chasiotis, D. (1983). The regulation of glycogen phosphorylase and glycogen breakdown in human skeletal muscle. *Acta Physiol. Scand.* (Suppl. 518), 1-68.

Chasiotis, D., & Hultman, E. (1985). The effect of adrenalin infusion on the regulation of glycogenolysis in human muscle during isometric contraction. *Acta Physiol. Scand.*, **123**, 55-60.

Chasiotis, D., Sahlin, K., & Hultman, E. (1983). Regulation of glycogenolysis in human muscle in response to epinephrine infusion. *J. Appl. Physiol.*, **54**, 45-50.

Cohen, P. (1980). The role of calcium ions, calmodulin and troponin in the regulation of phosphorylase kinase from rabbit skeletal muscle. *Eur. J. Biochem.*, **111**, 563-574.

Cohen, P. (1981). The role of calmodulin, troponin and cyclic AMP in the regulation of glycogen metabolism in mammalian skeletal muscle. *Adv. Cycl. Nucleot. Res.*, **14**, 345-359.

Constable, S.H., Favier, R.J., & Holloszy, J.O. (1986). Exercise and glycogen depletion: Effects on ability to activate muscle phosphorylase. *J. Appl. Physiol.*, **60**, 1518-1523.

Entman, M.L., Keslensky, S.S., Chu, A., & Van Winkle, W.B. (1980). The sarcoplasmic reticulum-glycogenolytic complex in mammalian fast twitch skeletal muscle. *J. Biol. Chem.*, **255**, 6245-6252.

Gollnick, P.D., Armstron, R.B., Semobrowich, W.L., Shepherd, E.E., & Saltin, B. (1973). Glycogen depletion pattern in human skeletal muscle fibers after heavy exercise. *J. Appl. Physiol.*, **34**, 615-618.

Harris, R.C., Bergström, J., & Hultman, E. (1971). The effect of propranolol on glycogen metabolism during exercise. In Pernow & B. Saltin (Eds.), *Muscle metabolism during exercise. Adv. Exp. Med. Biol. No. 11.* Plenum Press, New York-London, 301-305.

Hermansen, L., & Vaage, O. (1977). Lactate disappearance and glycogen synthesis in human muscle after maximal exercise. *Am. J. Physiol.*, **233**, E422-E429.

Huang, H., & Glinsman, W.H. (1976). Separation and characterization of two phosphorylase phosphatase inhibitors from rabbit skeletal muscle. *Eur. J. Biochem.*, **70**, 419-426.

Hultman, E. (1986). Carbohydrate metabolism during hard exercise and in the recovery period after exercise. *Acta Physiol. Scand.*, **556** (Suppl. 128), 75-82.

Hultman, E., & Bergström, J. (1973). Local energy-supplying substrates as limiting factors in different types of leg muscle work in normal man. In Keul (Ed.), *Limiting factors of physical performance.* Int. Symp. at Gravenbruch, 1971, Georg Thieme, Stuttgart, 113-125.

Hultman, E., & Sjöholm, H. (1983a). Substrate availability. In Knuttgen, Vogel, & Poortmans (Eds.), *Int. series on sport sciences, vol 13, biochemistry of exercise.* Human Kinetics, Champaign, IL, 63-75.

Hultman, E., & Sjöholm, H. (1983b). Engergy metabolism and contraction force of human skeletal muscle *in situ* during electrical stimulation. *J. Physiol.*, **345**, 525-532.

Hultman, E., & Sjöholm, H. (1986). Biochemical causes of fatigue. In Jones, McCartney, & McComas (Eds.), *Human muscle power.* Human Kinetics, Champaign, IL, 215-238.

Hultman, E., & Spriet, L.L. (1986). Skeletal muscle metabolism, contraction force and glycogen utilization during prolonged electrical stimulation in humans. *J. Physiol.*, **374**, 493-501.

Krebs, E.G., Love, D.S., Bratvold, G.E., Trayser, K.A., Meyer, W.L., & Fisher, E.H. (1964). Purification and properties of rabbit skeletal muscle phosphorylase *b* kinase. *Biochem.*, **3**, 1022-1033.

McGilvery, R.W. (1975). The use of fuels for muscular work. In Howald, & Poortmans (Eds.), *Metabolic adaptation to prolonged physical exercise.* Birkhäuser Verlag, Basel, 12-30.

Meyer, F., Heilmeyer, L.M.G., Haschke, R.H., & Fischer, E.H. (1970). Control of phosphorylase activity in a muscle glycogen particle. I. Isolation and characterization of the protein-glycogen complex. *J. Biol. Chem.*, **245**, 6642-6648.

Perry, S.V. (1974). Calcium ions and the functions of the contractile proteins of the muscle. *Biochem. Soc. Symp.*, **39**, 115.

Richter, E.A., Ruderman, N.B., Gavras, H., Belur, E.R., & Galbo, H. (1982). Muscle glycogenolysis during exercise: Dual control by epinephrine and contractions. *Am. J. Physiol.*, **242**, E25-E32.

Spriet, L.L., Ren, J.M., & Hultman, E. (1987). Human muscle glycogenolysis and force production during electrical stimulation and epinephrine infusion. *Med. Sci. Sports Exerc.*, **19** (Suppl. 2), S54.

Fatigue and the ATP Consuming and Producing Capacities of Muscle

P.D. Gollnick, D.R. Hodgson, L.A. Bertocci, E.H. Witt, and J. Chen

College of Veterinary Medicine, Washington State University, Pullman

During exercise a point is reached where its intensity must either be reduced or it must be terminated. That is, a point of fatigue or exhaustion is reached. Numerous factors are probably involved in establishing the point of the onset of fatigue or exhaustion, including depletion of intramuscular fuels, declines in pH, elevations in temperature, and dehydration. Under some exercise conditions, for example, high intensity exercise, the [ATP] of muscle declines. This demonstrates that muscle has a capacity to break down ATP more rapidly than it can be synthesized. The focus of this paper is on the relationships between the capacities for ATP use and production as they co-exist in muscle and are used during high-intensity exercise. Suggestions are made as to possible reasons for the onset of fatigue during heavy exercise.

Maximum Rate of ATP Hydrolysis During Muscular Contraction

The capacity of muscle to break down ATP can be estimated by several methods. One approach is to electrically stimulate muscle with the circulation occluded, thereby producing a closed system where the changes in high-energy phosphate ($\sim$P) can be estimated. In such closed systems declines in ATP and phosphocreatine (PC) concentrations and increased concentrations of lactate and other glycolytic intermediates involved in ATP production can be measured. To assess the maximum capacity for ATP hydrolysis during muscular contraction, changes must be measured before declines in muscular tension occur, that is, during the first seconds of the contraction. Kushmerick (1983) has summarized results from such experiments conducted on frog and mouse muscle. When data from mouse muscle are adjusted to 37° C, the maximal rates of ATP hydrolysis can be estimated to be 13.6 and 4.4 μmol of $\sim$P $\cdot$ g $\cdot$ s^{-1}, respectively, for the fast twitch extensor digitorium longus and slow twitch soleus muscles. When contractile activity was sustained beyond about 6 s, the rate of ATP hydrolysis of the extensor digitorium longus muscle declined to about 10% (1.2 μmol of $\sim$P $\cdot$ g $\cdot$ s^{-1}) of the peak rate. This value is similar to the rate of ATP hydrolysis (about 2.5 μmol of $\sim$P $\cdot$ g $\cdot$ s^{-1}) that occurs during electrical stimulation of rat muscle (Dudley & Terjung, 1985) and during short, heavy voluntary exercise performed by humans (Boobis et al., 1982; Cheetham et al., 1987). Thus during steady-state exercise the capacity for ATP hydrolysis is about one-fifth of the peak value.

ATP-Producing Capacity of Muscle

The principal ways for replenishing the ATP that is hydrolyzed during muscular contraction are via (a) transfer of $\sim P$ from PC to ADP, (b) lactate production, (c) terminal oxidation of fuels to CO_2 and H_2O, and (d) the adenylate kinase reaction. The maximal capacities of these systems can be estimated from the activities of key enzymes in the respective pathways and from actual values measured under conditions intended to produce maximal activation of each system.

Estimation of maximum rates of substrate flux through metabolic pathways based on selected enzyme rates runs the risk of using values for the maximal rates of enzymes that are measured under nonphysiological conditions of substrate and co-factor(s) concentrations, pH, temperature, and cellular organization. Most often the only objective is to find the maximum velocity (Vmax) of an enzyme-mediated reaction regardless of what conditions are required to produce it and without an attempt to determine the physiological meaning of the results that are generated. Although fully cognizant of the pitfalls of the method, we will make some estimates of ATP-producing capacity of muscle based on reported Vmax of selected enzymes. Here it has been assumed that the maximal rates that occur in tissue are one-half of the Vmax measured in vitro. This rate is at the Km for their respective substrates. To exceed this rate for multiple step pathways would require the maintenance of intracellular substrates at concentrations that would create unacceptable osmotic pressures (see Saltin & Gollnick, 1983).

The transfer of $\sim P$ from PC to ADP to form ATP is very rapid and prevents a fall in ATP under most conditions. This rapid transfer is possible due to the high activity of creatine phosphokinase, which averages approximately 20 $\mu mol \cdot g \cdot s^{-1}$ in most skeletal muscle (Staudte et al., 1973). At a rate of 50% of maximal, this would transfer about 10 μmol of $\sim P \cdot g \cdot s^{-1}$. At this rate the PC stored in muscle would be reduced to zero in a few seconds.

The capacities of the metabolic pathways can also be estimated from the Vmax of enzymes such as phosphorylase and phosphofructokinase of the Embden-Meyerhof pathway. On this basis, the maximum rate of substrate flux through this pathway would result in the generation of approximately 1.5 μmol of $\sim P \cdot g \cdot s^{-1}$ from the lactate produced. Based on the Vmax of citrate synthase, the $\sim P$ production for terminal oxidation could be as high as 9 $\mu mol \cdot g \cdot s^{-1}$. Thus, when considered only on the basis of flux through a single enzyme step, the capacity of muscle to generate ATP would appear to be present in excess.

Estimates of the capacity of muscle to consume oxygen based on the uptake of oxygen by muscle homogenates or isolated mitochondria have produced values ranging from 12 to 296 $ml \cdot kg \cdot min^{-1}$ (Davies et al., 1981; Holloszy, 1967). The highest of these rates is below that measured under in vivo conditions of voluntary exercise (Andersen & Saltin, 1985) where it is unlikely all of the muscle was fully activated and where a maximal value was not demonstrated by the classical plateauing of the oxygen uptake in response to an increase in power output. These inordinately low values from in vitro studies are probably due to destruction and/or loss of mitochondria during homogenization and isolation.

The capacity of the metabolic pathways to generate $\sim P$ may best be estimated from peak rates of lactate production and oxygen uptake by muscle. The maximal rate of lactate production appears to be about 0.50 $\mu mol \cdot g \cdot s^{-1}$. The maximum lactate concentration that can accumulate in muscle appears to range between 25 and 50 $\mu mol \cdot g^{-1}$, which is attained in about 90 s during maximal efforts. Thus maximal rates of lactate production would generate about 0.6 μmol of $\sim P \cdot g \cdot s^{-1}$. This rate of lactate production would contribute between 37.5 and 75 $\mu mol \cdot g^{-1}$ of $\sim P$ during a 90 s period of high-intensity exercise. The maximal reported rate of oxygen uptake is about 350 $ml \cdot kg \cdot min^{-1}$ (5.8 $\mu l \cdot g \cdot s^{-1}$) (Andersen & Saltin, 1985). This is equivalent to a $\sim P$ production of 1.55 $\mu mol \cdot g \cdot s^{-1}$.

ATP can be produced by the adenylate kinase reaction where $2\ ADP \rightleftharpoons ATP + AMP$. The amount of ATP generated via this reaction is difficult to assess directly. An indirect indication can be obtained from the accumulation of NH_4 in the muscle, as this appears to be linked to adenosine monophosphate formation via deamination of inosine monophosphate. From the kinetics of NH_4 accumulation in electrically stimulated muscle it does not appear that this is an important source of ATP until lactate accumulation plateaus, and then only about 4 μmol of $NH_4 \cdot g^{-1}$ wet muscle accumulated (Dudley & Terjung, 1985). This would represent a relatively small contribution to the total ATP turnover of muscle. However, it could be important in times of severe exercise where the total ATP content of the muscle declines (see Table 1).

Table 1   Summary of the Potential and Actual ATP-Consuming and Producing Capacity of Muscle

	μmol $\cdot$ g $\cdot$ s^{-1}
ATP-splitting capacity	
Sustainable rate in man	2.5
ATP-producing capacity	
Estimated from enzyme activities*	
Creatine kinase	10
Citrate synthase	9
Phosphofructokinase	9
From measured values in muscle	
Lactate production	0.6
Oxygen uptake	1.5

Note. *Estimates are based on enzyme activities adjusted to 37 °C and 50% of the Vmax being the peak in vivo rate (see text).

Effect of Exercise on ATP Concentration of Muscle

Although there were earlier reports of declines in [ATP] following electrical stimulation (e.g., Helmreich & Cori, 1964), Hultman and co-workers (1967) were perhaps the first to observe declines in [ATP] in human skeletal muscle after voluntary exercise. They reported a 40% reduction in [ATP] following 1 to 2 min of heavy exercise. Karlsson and Saltin (1971) observed a similar decline after several bouts of high intensity exercise. Since then there have been numerous reports of decrements in the [ATP] of muscle following either spontaneous exercise or electrical stimulation.

Responses of the Metabolic Pathways to Exercise

Oxygen Delivery

From the above it is clear that muscle possesses a high capacity for ATP turnover and that at times there is a mismatch between ATP breakdown and resynthesis. The major purpose of this paper is to address the question of why this mismatch occurs when the capacity for ATP production appears to be so high. One factor that has been examined in fairly great detail is the capacity of the circulatory system to deliver oxygen to the muscle and then the ability of the muscle to use the oxygen presented to it. The most significant recent revelations regarding the circulatory response to exercise have come from the studies of Andersen and Saltin (1985) where the blood flow and oxygen uptake of a small muscle group were measured. This study, along with the work of Rowell et al. (1986), suggested that the capacity of the local circulation to accept blood flow has not yet been measured. These data suggest that during activity that engages a large muscle mass, the limiting factor is the ability to deliver blood to the working muscle and that this is probably limited by the capacity of the heart to pump adequate volumes of blood. During such exercise changes occur in muscle that appear to modify its capacity to generate ATP. These changes are addressed at this time.

Lactate Production and pH

It is well known that with heavy exercise there is a large production of lactate and that this lactate accumulates in both muscle and blood, resulting in declines in their pHs. Thus, there are numerous reports that the pH of skeletal muscle falls to between 6.2 and 6.4 during heavy exercise (Hermansen & Osnes, 1972; Sahlin et al., 1976), with a few reports of values as low as 6.0 (Taylor et al., 1986). The potential effect of such reductions in pH on the function of several systems within muscle have been summarized by Mainwood and Renaud (1985). Since enzyme activities are influenced by pH, it was logical to examine the effects of pH on the activities of key enzymes. Perhaps the most cited study regarding the effect of pH on an enzyme rate is that of Trivedi and Danforth (1966) where it was reported that the phosphofructokinase activity of frog muscle was nearly zero at pH 7.1. This has been widely accepted as indicating that the decline in the pH of muscle occurring during strenuous exercise effectively inhibits further lactate production by the inhibition of this key enzyme of the Embden-Meyerhof pathway.

However, these results must be evaluated carefully when applied to intact muscle. The importance of this pH effect on phosphofructokinase must be considered with knowledge that the pH of resting muscle may be less than 7.1, and this would appear to preclude the formation of any lactate. Furthermore, there are innumerable reports of a continued production by and accumulation of lactate in muscle where the pH is below 6.6. These data demonstrate that the results from homogenates of frog muscle cannot be universally applied to the intact muscle, mammalian or other. Thus, either conditions exist within muscle that protect the enzyme from inactivation at a relatively low pH and high lactate concentration, or species differences exist. The recent report of Dobson et al. (1986) presents data that suggest that conditions exist within muscle to protect against the pH-induced inactivation of phosphofructokinase. However, at the very low pHs that have been reported, it is likely that some inhibition of enzyme does occur.

Aerobic Metabolism and pH

A number of reports have suggested that structural damage may occur in mitochondria after exercise (Gollnick et al., 1971; Gollnick & King, 1969; Laugens & Gomez-Dumm, 1967; Nimmo & Snow, 1982; Warhol et al., 1985). There are also reports that the yield of mitochondria from skeletal muscle and their respiratory capacity are lower after exercise (Davies et al., 1982; Dohm et al., 1972, 1975). In contrast to these are reports that the ultrastructural changes seen after exercise are artifacts of the fixation methods (Bowers et al., 1974) and that the respiratory function of mitochondria is not altered by exercise (Terjung et al., 1972). Subsequent reports have suggested that the basis for the structural and functional changes that occur in mitochondria following exercise may be linked either to oxygen free radical accumulation in muscle (Davies et al., 1982) or in liver to excessive increases in free fatty acids (Klug et al., 1984).

The reduction in intramuscular pH that occurs in conjunction with elevations in lactate could alter mitochondrial function. This possibility is supported by in vitro studies. For example, Hansford (1972) observed that the uptake of oxygen by mitochondria at pH 6.4 was only 45% of the peak value. Armiger et al. (1974) have observed structural changes in mitochondria following in vitro incubation with lactate concentrations similar to those that exist in muscle following strenuous exercise.

Klug et al. (1984) have observed decrements in the function mitochondria isolated from rat liver following exhaustive exercise. This was associated with elevations in free fatty acids and could be reversed by incubation of mitochondria with albumin, which removes fatty acids from mitochondria. Incubation of isolated mitochondria with palmitate produced a dose-dependent loss of respiratory capacity and also resulted in a loss of mitochondrial-bound hexokinase.

Based on the previous findings of changes in mitochondrial oxidation at low pH, we (Bertocci & Gollnick, 1985; Witt et al., 1987) measured the respiratory capacity of muscle following multiple bouts of supramaximal exercise that lowered the pH of muscle and blood due to production and accumulation of lactate in these tissues. These data demonstrated that the respiratory capacity of mitochondria fell to about 50% of the rest value when muscle pH was 6.4. This value is similar to the suppression in respiratory capacity reported by Hansford (1972) following the in vitro incubation of mitochondria at pH 6.4. Respiratory capacity had returned to near the control value 60 min post-exercise, by which time muscle pH was also normal. In these studies we took great care to avoid destruction of mitochondria. Precautions taken included limiting the number of passes of the pestle during homogenization (Bertocci & Gollnick, 1985) and the use of trypsin to release mitochondria from muscle samples without homogenization (Witt et al., 1987).

Although declines in the respiratory capacity of mitochondria are associated with declines in pH, it cannot be assumed that this is the only intracellular change responsible for the post-exercise effect. Thus, the loss of mitochondrial-bound hexokinase could be involved in the loss of oxidative capacity. Support for the concept that a reduction in mitochondrial function may be linked to a loss of mitochondrial-bound hexokinase comes from the observation that treatment of isolated mitochondria with palmitate resulted in a loss of mitochondrial-bound hexokinase (Klug et al., 1984). A reduction in mitochondrial-bound hexokinase can also be produced by elevations in the concentration glucose-6-PO_4 (Rose & Warms, 1967). In preliminary studies Chen et al. (1987) observed that the fraction of mitochondrial-bound hexokinase was reduced to nearly zero following heavy exercise. The extent of the reduction in mitochondrial-bound hexokinase was correlated to an elevation in glucose-6-PO_4 concentration in muscle following exercise. It was also associated with a loss of respiratory capacity both in muscle samples obtained following supramaximal exercise and in isolated mitochondria in an in vitro incubation with glucose-6-PO_4 concentrations similar to those that existed in the muscle following exercise.

Significance of Depressions in Respiratory Capacity of Mitochondria

A question that must be asked concerns the significance of the reduction in the respiratory capacity of mitochondria as it relates to the function of the muscle and of the whole body to exercise. Clearly, the oxygen uptake of humans does not decline during heavy exercise when the pH of muscle is low. This suggests that the decline in respiratory capacity of skeletal muscle observed in in vitro analysis may not occur in vivo. However, this is probably not the case since large-muscle activity that results in the attainment of total-body maximal oxygen uptake does not require the engagement of the entire muscle mass. Even with exercise such as cycle ergometry, the mass of muscle engaged is less than that available. Thus, during the course of activity, some motor units could become inactive and others that were initially inactive could be recruited. This would allow the exercise to continue and total body oxygen uptake to remain high. This type of progressive recruitment of motor units has been demonstrated during moderately severe prolonged exercise (Gollnick et al., 1973).

Summary

An analysis of existing data reveals that under conditions of heavy exercise there is a decline in the ATP content of skeletal muscle. This has been linked to changes in the functional capacity of mitochondria. Evidence does exist that suggests that ultrastructural changes may occur in mitochondria following a variety of types and intensities of exercise. These changes in structure and function have been linked to the production of oxygen free radicals and to elevations in free fatty acids in the liver. Evidence is presented suggesting that these changes may also be the result of decreases in pH and of elevations in glucose-6-PO_4 concentrations that release mitochondrial-bound hexokinase.

Acknowledgments

Supported in part by grants from the Washington State Equine Research Program.

References

Andersen, P., & Saltin, B. (1985). Maximal perfusion of skeletal muscle in man. *J. Physiol. (London)*, **366**, 233-249.

Armiger, L., Gavin, J.B., & Herdson, P.B. (1974). Mitochondrial changes in dog myocardium induced by neutral lactate *in vitro*. *Lab. Invest.*, **31**, 29-33.

Bertocci, L.A., & Gollnick, P.D. (1985). pH effect on mitochondria and individual enzyme function. *Med. Sci. Sports Exer.*, **17**, 259.

Boobis, L., Williams, C., & Wootton, S.A. (1982). Human muscle metabolism during brief maximal exercise. *J. Physiol. (London)*, **338**, 21-22P.

Bowers, W.R. Jr., Hubbard, R.W., Smoake, J.A., Daum, R.C., & Nilson, E. (1974). Effects of exercise on the ultrastructure of skeletal muscle. *Am. J. Physiol.*, **227**, 313-316.

Cheetham, M.E., Boobis, L.H., Brooks, S., & Williams, C. (1986). Human muscle metabolism during sprint running. *J. Appl. Physiol.*, **61**, 54-60.

Chen, J., Hodgson, D.R., Rose, R.J., & Gollnick, P.D. (1987). Effect of exercise on the fraction of mitochondrial bound hexokinase of skeletal muscle. *Med. Sci. Sports Exer.*, **19**, S81.

Davies, K.J.A., Packer, L., & Brooks, G.A. (1981). Biochemical adaptations of mitochondria, muscle, and whole-body respiration to endurance training. *Arch. Biochem. Biophys.*, **209**, 539-554.

Davies, K.J.A., Quintanilha, A.T., Brooks, G.A., & Packer, L. (1982). Free radicals and tissue damage produced by exercise. *Biochem. Biophys. Res. Comm.*, **104**, 1198-1205.

Dobson, G.P., Yamamota, E., & Hochachka, P.W. (1986). Phosphofructokinase control in muscle: Nature and reversal of pH-dependent ATP inhibition. *Am. J. Physiol.*, **250**, R71-R76.

Dohm, G.L., Barakat, H., Stephensen, T.P., Pennington, S.N., & Tapscott, E.B. (1975). Changes in muscle mitochondrial lipid composition resulting from training and exhaustive exercise. *Life Sci.*, **17**, 1075-1080.

Dohm, G.L., Huston, R.L., Askew, E.W., & Weiser, P.C. (1972). Effects of exercise on activity of heart and muscle mitochondria. *Am. J. Physiol.*, **223**, 783-787.

Dudley, G.A., & Terjung, R.L. (1985). Influence of aerobic metabolism on IMP accumulation in fast-twitch muscle. *Am. J. Physiol.*, **248**, C37-C42.

Gollnick, P.D., & King, W.D. (1969). Effect of exercise and training on mitochondria of rat skeletal muscle. *Am. J. Physiol.*, **216**, 1502-1509.

Gollnick, P.D., Ianuzzo, C.D., & King, D.W. (1971). Ultrastructural and enzyme changes in muscles with exercise. In B. Pernow & B. Saltin (Eds.), *Muscle metabolism during exercise*. New York, Plenum, 69-85.

Hansford, R.G. (1972). Some properties of pyruvate and 2-oxoglutarate oxidation by blowfly flight-muscle mitochondria. *Biochem. J.*, **127**, 271-283.

Helmreich, E., & Cori, C.F. (1964). Regulation of glycolysis in muscle. *Advan. Enz. Reg.*, **3**, 91-107.

Hermansen, L., & Osnes, J. (1972). Blood and muscle pH after maximal exercise in man. *J. Appl. Physiol.*, **32**, 304-308.

Holloszy, J.O. (1967). Biochemical adaptations in muscle. Effects of exercise on mitochondrial oxygen uptake and respiratory enzyme activity in skeletal muscle. *J. Biol. Chem.*, **242**, 2278-2282.

Hultman, E., Bergström, J., & McLennan-Anderson, N. (1967). Breakdown and resynthesis of phosphorylcreatine and adenosine triphosphate in connection with muscular work in man. *Scand. J. Clin. Lab. Invest.*, **19**, 56-66.

Karlsson, J., & Saltin, B. (1971). Oxygen deficit and muscle metabolites in intermittent exercise. *Acta Physiol. Scand.*, **82**, 115-122.

Klug, G., Krause, A.J., Östlund, A-K., Knoll, G., & Brdiczka, D. (1984). Alteration in liver mitochondrial function as a result of fasting and exhaustive exercise. *Biochim. Biophys. Acta.*, **764**, 272-282.

Kushmerick, M.J. (1983). Energetics of muscle contraction. In L.D. Peachy, R.H. Ardrian, & S.R. Geiger (Eds.), *Handbook of Physiology-Skeletal Muscle*. Williams & Wilkins, Baltimore, 189-235.

Laugens, R., & Gomez-Dumm, C.L.A. (1967). Fine structure of myocardial mitochondria in rats after exercise for one-half to two-hours. *Circulation Res.*, **21**, 271-279.

Mainwood, G.W., & Renaud, J.M. (1985). The effect of acid-base balance on fatigue of skeletal muscle. *Can. J. Physiol. Pharmacol.*, **63**, 403-416.

Nimmo, M.A., & Snow, D.H. (1982). Time course of ultrastructural changes in skeletal muscle after two types of exercise. *J. Appl. Physiol.*, **52**, 910-913.

Rose, I.W., & Warms, J.W.B. (1967). Mitochondrial hexokinase: Release, rebinding, and location. *J. Biol. Chem.*, **242**, 1635-1645.

Rowell, L.B., Saltin, B., Kiens, B., & Christensen, N.J. (1986). Is peak quadriceps blood flow in humans even higher during exercise with hypoxemia? *Am. J. Physiol.*, **251**, H1038-H1044.

Sahlin, K., Harris, R.C., Nylind, B., & Hultman, E. (1976). Lactate content and pH in muscle samples obtained after dynamic exercise. *Pflügers Arch.*, **367**, 143-149.

Saltin, B., & Gollnick, P.D. (1983). Skeletal muscle adaptability: Significance for metabolism and performance. In L.D. Peachy, R.H. Ardrian, & S.R. Geiger (Eds.), *Handbook of Physiology-Skeletal Muscle*. Williams & Wilkins, Baltimore, 555-631.

Staudte, H., Exner, G.U., & Pette, D. (1973). Effects of short-term high intensity (sprint) training on some contractile and metabolic characteristics of fast and slow muscle of the rat. *Pflügers Arch.*, **344**, 159-168.

Taylor, D.G., Styles, P., Matthews, P.M., Arnold, D.A., Gadian, D.G., Bore, P., & Radda, G.K. (1986). Energetics of human muscle: Exercise-induced ATP depletion. *Magn. Res. Med.*, **3**, 44-54.

Terjung, R.L., Baldwin, K.M., Molé, P.A., Klinkerfuss, G.H., & Holloszy J.O. (1972). Effect of running to exhaustion on skeletal muscle mitochondria: A biochemical study. *Am. J. Physiol.*, **223**, 549-554.

Trivedi, B., & Danforth, W.H. (1966). Effect of pH on the kinetics of frog muscle phosphofructokinase. *J. Biol. Chem.*, **241**, 4110-4112.

Warhol, M.J., Siegel, A.J., Evans, W.J., & Silverman, L.M. (1985). Skeletal muscle injury and repair in marathon runners after competition. *Am. J. Pathol.*, **118**, 331-339.

Witt, E.H., Kelso, T.B., McCutcheon, L.J., Rose, R.J., Hodgson, D.R., & Gollnick, P.D. (1987). Effect of maximal exercise on mitochondrial respiratory and citrate synthase activity. *Med. Sci. Sports Exer.*, **19**, S43.

Lactate Formulation During Submaximal Exercise Is Oxygen Dependent

K. Sahlin and A. Katz

Department of Clinical Physiology, Karolinska Institute, Huddinge University Hospital, Stockholm, Sweden

Berzelius discovered lactate (La) in exercised muscle in 1841 (see du Bois-Reymond, 1877), and since then, it has been a metabolite of central importance in exercise physiology. The reason for this is the close connection between La formation and muscle fatigue. Formation of La is associated with a stoichiometric formation of H^+ and several metabolic and contractile processes are known to be negatively affected by a decrease in pH (see Hermansen, 1981), which could thereby explain the connection between muscle fatigue and La accumulation at high exercise intensities (Hermansen, 1981; Sahlin, 1986). La, however, is also formed during submaximal exercise, and the exercise intensity where the breakpoint between aerobic and anaerobic ATP production occurs has been termed the lactate threshold. The lactate threshold is closely related to performance during long-distance running (Sjödin & Jacobs, 1981). This is probably related to the accelerated rate of glycolysis and La formation that occurs at and above this exercise intensity. This indicates also a rapid loss of glycogen within the working muscle, which has been associated with muscle fatigue.

The reason for La formation at submaximal exercise is not fully understood. The hypothesis that La formation is due to an inadequate O_2 availability in the contracting muscle is supported by findings that submaximal exercise during inspiration of a gas with a decreased fraction of O_2 results in increased muscle (Linnarsson et al., 1974) and blood (Hughes et al., 1968) La concentrations compared with normoxic exercise. Recent studies have, however, shown that the O_2 tension (PO_2) within an La-producing, contracting muscle is above the level where cellular respiration is diminished (Connett et al., 1984), and from these findings it was concluded that La production during submaximal exercise was not due to hypoxia (Brooks, 1985; Connett et al., 1984). A part of the apparent controversy exists because hypoxia at the cellular level could be defined in at least two ways (a) cellular respiration is affected by PO_2, and (b) cellular metabolism is affected by PO_2. This report will focus on the questions of how cellular metabolism is affected by a decreased O_2 availability, and why this occurs before cellular respiration is affected.

Muscle NADH Content and O_2 Availability

A decreased O_2 availability at the mitochondrial level will result in a reduction of the mitochondrial NAD^+ to NADH ratio. An increase of mitochondrial NADH is therefore a sensitive index of the O_2 availability in the mitochondria (Chance, 1976). The muscle content of NADH will include NADH from all cellular compartments. Data from cyanide-poisoned (Sahlin & Katz, 1986) and ischaemic (Sahlin, 1983) muscle, however, support the notion that changes in whole-muscle NADH primarily reflect changes within the mitochondria. Changes in total muscle NADH will therefore give information about changes in the mitochondrial redox state and could be used as an index of the O_2 availability at the mitochondrial level.

Effect of Respiratory Hypoxia on Muscle NADH and La Formation

Eight men cycled for 5 min at 120 $\pm$ 6 watts ($\overline{X}$ $\pm$ SE), at which O_2 uptake was 50% of their maximal O_2 uptake, breathing room air (21% O_2; normoxia) on one occasion and 11% O_2 in N_2 (resp. hypoxia) on the other. Biopsies from the quadriceps femoris muscle and arterial blood samples were obtained before and after exercise. Further details of the experimental procedure and the analytical methods are available elsewhere (Katz & Sahlin, 1987).

Oxygen uptake during exercise was not significantly different between resp. hypoxia (1.59 $\pm$ 0.08 L/min) and normoxia (1.55 $\pm$ 0.08). Muscle NADH content was similar at rest under both conditions but was significantly higher ($p < .01$) after exercise during resp. hypoxia vs. normoxia (Table 1). Exercise during resp. hypoxia also resulted in a higher muscle and blood La content and a lower PCr content in muscle (Table 1). In skeletal muscle creatine kinase reaction is considered to be close to equilibrium, and a decrease in PCr will therefore occur when either ADP or H^+ are increased (Figure 1). A decrease in PCr will also result in an increase in inorganic phosphate (P_i) (Figure 1).

Table 1   Muscle Metabolites (mmol/kg d.wt.) and Blood La (mmol/L) at Rest and After 5 Min of Exercise at 120 W

	Rest		Exercise	
	Normoxia	Resp. hx	Normoxia	Resp. hx
NADH	0.136 $\pm$ 0.018	0.144 $\pm$ 0.018	0.117 $\pm$ 0.008	0.172 $\pm$ 0.014**
La	1.8 $\pm$ 0.5	1.7 $\pm$ 0.4	8.6 $\pm$ 1.0	33.2 $\pm$ 5.2**
PCr	77.1 $\pm$ 1.3	78.5 $\pm$ 2.3	53.5 $\pm$ 2.8	42.4 $\pm$ 3.7*
ATP	24.3 $\pm$ 0.6	24.8 $\pm$ 0.6	24.0 $\pm$ 0.7	24.6 $\pm$ 0.6
Blood La	0.7 $\pm$ 0.2	0.7 $\pm$ 0.1	2.3 $\pm$ 0.1	6.0 $\pm$ 0.5***

Note. Values are means $\pm$ *SE* and are from Katz & Sahlin (1987).
$*p < .05$; $**p < .01$; $***p < .001$ resp. hx vs. normoxia.

$$PCr \ + \ ADP \ + \ n_1H^+ \ \longleftrightarrow \ Cr \ + \ ATP$$

$$ATP \ \longrightarrow \ ADP \ + \ Pi \ + \ n_2H^+$$

$$\text{net reaction: } PCr \ + \ n_3H^+ \ \longrightarrow \ Cr \ + \ Pi$$

Figure 1.   The creatine kinase and ATPase reactions. Values for n_1, n_2 and n_3 are $\leqslant 1$ and are dependent on pH and the concentration of Mg^{2+}.

Metabolic Changes and Cellular Respiration

Evidence is available that the first two phosphorylation sites in the respiratory chain are close to equilibrium (see Wilson et al., 1977). A theoretical formula has been derived by Kushmerick (1983) to describe the dependence of cellular respiration (VO_2) on PO_2, the mitochondrial redox state, and the phosphorylation potential (Figure 2). From this formula it is evident that an increased VO_2 can be achieved by an increase in NADH, ADP, or P_i. Exercise during resp. hypoxia results in a decreased PO_2 in arterial blood (Katz & Sahlin, 1987) and will probably cause a decreased PO_2 in the working muscle as compared to normoxia. However, VO_2 was maintained during resp. hypoxia, and the increases in NADH, ADP, and P_i (decreased PCr content) during resp. hypoxia could therefore be regarded as metabolic adaptations, which primarily serve to activate the aerobic ATP production. The increase in ADP will result in increased AMP values (via the adenylate kinase reaction), which in addition to the higher P_i values will activate glycogenolysis (Chasiotis & Start, 1983; Newsholme & Start, 1973) and glycolysis (Newsholme, 1973). An accelerated glycolysis, together with an elevated cytosolic redox state (Katz & Sahlin, 1987), will result in an increased La formation.

$$\dot{V}O_2 = k \times PO_2 \times \left(\frac{NADH}{NAD}\right)^{\frac{1}{2}} \times \left(\frac{ADP \times P_i}{ATP}\right)^{\frac{3}{2}}$$

Figure 2. Theoretical formula for regulation of oxygen consumption. For further details, see Kushmerick (1983).

Conclusion

It is concluded that inspiration of a gas with a low fraction of O_2 during exercise induces an increased content of NADH in muscle. Indirect evidence indicates that the increase in NADH occurs within the mitochondria, which therefore reflects a relative lack of O_2 at the cellular level. In a previous study we observed a decrease of NADH (and no change in La) during low-intensity exercise (40% $\dot{V}O_2$max) and an increase of NADH and lactate above the values at rest when the exercise intensity was increased to 75% and 100% $\dot{V}O_2$max (Sahlin et al., 1987). These data, together with the present findings, suggest that La production during normoxic submaximal exercise is O_2-dependent.

Acknowledgments

This study was supported by grants from the Swedish Sports Research Council and the Swedish Medical Research Council (No. 7670). A. Katz was the recipient of a fellowship from the Swedish Institute.

References

Bois-Reymond, du, E. (1877). Uber angeblich saure Reaction des Muskelfleisches. In *Gesammelte Abhandl. zur allg. Muskel- u. Nervenphysik*, 2-36.

Brooks, G.A. (1985). Anaerobic threshold: Review of the concept and directions for future research. *Med. Sci. Sports Exer.*, **17**, 22-31.

Chance, B. (1976). Pyridine nucleotide as an indicator of the oxygen requirements for energy-linked functions of mitochondria. *Circulation Res.*, **38**(Suppl. 1) I31-I38.

Chasiotis, D. (1983). The regulation of glycogen phosphorylase and glycogen breakdown in human skeletal muscle. *Acta Physiol. Scand.*, (Suppl. 518).

Connett, R.J., Gayeski, T.E.J., & Honig, C.R. (1984). Lactate accumulation in fully aerobic, working dog gracilis muscle. *Am. J. Physiol.*, **246**, H120-H128.

Hermansen, L. (1981). Effect of metabolic changes on force generation in skeletal muscle during maximal exercise. In R. Porter & J. Whelan (Eds.), *Human muscle fatigue: Physiological mechanisms*. Pitman Medical, London, 75-88.

Hughes, R.L., Clode, M., Edwards, R.H.T., Godwin, T.J., & Jones, N.L. (1968). Effect of inspired O_2 on cardiopulmonary and metabolic responses to exercise. *J. Appl. Physiol.*, **2**, 336-347.

Katz, A., & Sahlin, K. (1987). Effect of decreased oxygen availability on NADH and lactate contents in human skeletal muscle during exercise. *Acta Physiol. Scand.*, **131**, 119-127.

Kushmerick, M.J. (1983). Energetics of muscle contraction. In L.D. Peachey, R.H. Adrian, & S.R. Greger (Eds.), *Skeletal muscle. Handbook of physiology 10*. Am. Physiol. Society, Bethesda, 189-236.

Linnarsson, D., Karlsson, J., Fagraeus, L., & Saltin, B. (1974). Muscle metabolites and oxygen deficit with exercise in hypoxia and hyperoxia. *J. Appl. Physiol.*, **36**, 399-402.

Newsholme, E., & Start, C. (1973). *Regulation in metabolism*. Wiley and Sons, England.

Sahlin, K. (1986). Muscle fatigue and lactic acid accumulation. *Acta Physiol. Scand.*, **128**(Suppl. 556), 83-91.

Sahlin, K. (1983). NADH and NADPH in human skeletal muscle at rest and during ischaemia. *Clin. Physiol.*, **3**, 477-485.

Sahlin, K., & Katz, A. (1986). The content of NADH in rat skeletal muscle at rest and after cyanide poisoning. *Biochem. J.*, **239**, 245-248.

Sahlin, K., Katz, A., & Henriksson, J. (1987). Redox state and lactate accumulation in human skeletal muscle during dynamic exercise. *Biochem. J.*, **245**, 551-556.

Sjödin, B., & Jacobs, I. (1981). Onset of blood lactate accumulation and marathon running performance. *Int. J. Sports Medicine.*, **2**, 23-26.

Wilson, D.F., Erecinska, M., Drown, C., & Silver, I.A. (1977). Effect of oxygen tension on cellular energetics. *Am. J. Physiol.*, **233**, C135-C140.

Elite Invertebrate Athletes: Flight in Insects, Its Metabolic Requirements and Regulation and Its Effects on Life Span

G. Wegener

Institut für Zoologie der Johannes Gutenberg-Universität, Mainz, G.F.R.

Exercise physiology has been restricted mainly to man and a few mammals. A comparative approach could provide new insight because special lifestyles often require particular mechanisms to be more clearly expressed in certain animals, while on the other hand, a fundamental similarity of life processes does exist. Hence, it may be worthwhile to look at animals that have extreme capabilities. Insects are, in this respect, a case in point, having developed all kinds of locomotion such as running, jumping, swimming, and flying, usually with very high efficiency. Most conspicuous is their ability to fly, and this has been extensively studied, while the other forms of locomotion have been rather neglected (Herreid & Fourtner, 1981; Herreid & Full, 1984).

In terms of energy, flight is the most expensive means of locomotion per unit of time, but it is much more economical when the distance traveled is taken into account (Tucker, 1973). This is reflected in the fact that some birds and insects migrate thousands of kilometers per year while small running animals do not.

To appreciate the physiological achievements insects have made, the main characteristics of their body organization should be mentioned: (a) Insects have an exoskeleton, consequently they grow discontinuously by molting and their final size is limited; (b) Insects have an open circulatory system and their organs are not capillarized; (c) Oxygen is conveyed to the tissues very efficiently by means of air-filled tubes, the tracheae; and (d) Insects are ectothermic, their body temperature can vary (to some extent without loss of function) depending on environmental conditions and/or metabolic rate.

Energy Metabolism of Insect Flight Muscle

Because of its great energy demand, active flight can only be sustained by aerobic ATP production. Hence, the metabolic demand of flight is, at any time, reliably reflected by oxygen consumption. Oxygen consumption can increase with the onset of flight up to 70-fold in locusts and more than a 100-fold in some other insects (for review, see Beenakkers et al., 1984; Kammer & Heinrich, 1978). Small mammals or birds, running or flying at maximum speed, would increase their respiration by only 7- to 14-fold. Considerations of this kind would bear more meaning if they could be based on active tissue. Flight muscle of a locust accounts for about 18% of body weight. The metabolic rate of resting flight muscle is not known. In humans the metabolic rate of skeletal muscle at rest is approximately 50% ($0.08 \ \mu\text{mol O}_2 \cdot \text{min}^{-1} \cdot \text{g}^{-1}$ muscle) of the basal metabolic rate ($0.16 \ \mu\text{mol O}_2 \cdot \text{min}^{-1} \cdot \text{g}^{-1}$ body mass). If the same relationship held true in locusts, ATP turnover in flight muscle would increase by nearly 800-fold at the onset of flight (Table 1), and this

Table 1   Oxygen Consumption and ATP Turnover Rates in Locusts at Rest and Flying at Maximum Speed

	Resting	Working	Working/Resting
O_2 consumption of locust in μmol per min and g body weight	0.47 (at 28 °C)	33[a]	70
(O_2 consumption of humans)	(0.16)	(3.2)	(20)
O_2 consumption in μmol per min per g flight muscle	0.235[b]	183.3[b]	780
(per g human skeletal muscle)	0.08	(6.4)	(80)
ATP turnover rates in μmol per s and g in flight muscle	0.0235[c]	18.3[c]	780
(in human skeletal muscle, aerobic)	(0.008)	(0.64)	(80)
(in human skeletal muscle, anaerobic)		(≤3)	
Contents of high energy phosphates in μmol per g muscle			
ATP, flight muscle[d]	5.05		
phosphoarginine	8.77		
(ATP, human skeletal muscle)	4.6		
(phosphocreatine, human skeletal muscle)	17.0		

Note. Corresponding data for humans at rest and during heavy muscular work are given in parentheses (for references, see Newsholme & Leech, 1983). [a]Maximum rate during initial phase of flight as estimated by Weis-Fogh (1952). [b]Based on the assumptions that the metabolic rate of resting muscle is 1/2 of the basal metabolic rate (see text), and that the increase in respiration upon flight is confined to the working flight muscle (about 18% of body mass) and not changed in other parts of the body. [c]For the sake of simplicity the rates have been calculated on the basis that all ATP is produced from the oxidation of carbohydrates (although fatty acids are a major fuel, at least for resting human muscle). With glucose as the sole substrate, the production of 1 mol of ATP is equivalent to the consumption of 6/36 = 0.16 mol of O_2. Contribution of lipid would decrease the ATP yield at a given O_2 consumption. If palmitate or tripalmitoylglycerol is oxidized, 1 mol of ATP is equivalent to 23/129 = 0.178, or 72.5/409 = 0.177 mol of O_2, respectively. [d]Rowan and Newsholme (1979).

would require corresponding increases in pathways like glycolysis, Krebs cycle, and respiratory chain. The problem is aggravated as very high rates of ATP hydrolysis are not matched by correspondingly high contents of energy-rich phosphates (see Table 1).

In insect flight muscle the phosphagen content is less than in mammalian skeletal muscle, although maximum ATP turnover rates are markedly higher in insect flight muscle than in mammalian muscle. Consequently, while the phosphagen content of human leg muscle could support contraction for about 5 seconds (for review, see Newsholme & Leech, 1983), the content of phosphoarginine (the phosphagen of insect) would be exhausted in less than 0.5 s in locust, and in less than 0.1 s in honeybee and blowfly muscle. However, ATP content of flight muscle does not change to a significant degree in working flight muscle. Therefore, ATP production must increase within a fraction of a second. In the locust, most of the muscle glycogen is degraded within 3 s of flight (Rowan & Newsholme, 1979). Utilization of glycogen requires a simultaneous activation of glycolysis, but how this is achieved is not known (neither for insect flight nor for vertebrate skeletal muscle). Phosphofructokinase (EC 2.7.1.11) is commonly regarded as an important enzyme in the regulation of glycolytic flux. Phosphofructokinase is strongly inhibited at physiological concentrations of ATP, and this inhibition can be removed in vitro by activators (deinhibitors). Phosphofructokinase purified from locust flight muscle is activated by NH_4^+, inorganic phosphate, AMP, and fructose 2,6-bisphosphate (Wegener et al., 1987a).

In view of the rapid activation of ATP turnover in insect flight muscle, it appeared desirable to measure tissue contents of inorganic phosphate and of high-energy phosphates under in vivo conditions. The nondestructive and noninvasive method of ^{31}P-NMR spectroscopy was therefore adapted to locust flight muscle. This demonstrated in resting muscle a much lower content of inorganic phosphate than would have been expected from biochemical analyses. Upon flight a marked decrease in the content of phosphoarginine and a concomitant increase in inorganic phosphate (that had also not been detectable in biochemical analyses) were seen (Wegener et al., 1987b).

Simulation of the phosphofructokinase reaction at near physiological concentrations of substrates, products, and effectors showed a more than 50-fold increase in enzyme activity when inorganic phosphate was increased from 1 to 5 mM. From these experiments the phosphagen system would appear to have an important activatory role, via inorganic phosphate, in addition to buffering the ATP concentration of the muscle cell. Inorganic phosphate stimulates the catabolism of carbohydrate at various steps: It is a substrate of glycogen phosphorylase and a potent activator of both hexokinase and phosphofructokinase. It is, however, still not clear whether the changes in the concentrations of known activators and their synergistic effects are sufficient to account for the increase in phosphofructokinase activity or whether additional mechanisms are recruited. Insect flight muscle seems to be a promising model to study this problem.

Flight muscles of many insects are designed not only for high energy output but also for sustained exercise and would show no fatigue unless their energy stores are depleted. Locusts in the field may fly from morning to dusk. In the laboratory they can be kept flying for many hours at an average metabolic rate of 5.25 J per g body weight per min, 25 times their basal metabolic rate (Weis-Fogh, 1952). Flight endurance in locusts is directly correlated with the amount of fat stored. In well-nourished locusts lipid stores should allow flight for up to 20 hours. Shortly after the onset of flight, fat replaces carbohydrate as the major fuel, although the carbohydrate stores are not depleted. Hence, oxidation of glucose must be inhibited, and much effort has been put into the elucidation of how this is achieved (for references, see Wegener et al., 1987a). Recently, the content of fructose 2,6-bisphosphate has been reported to fall in flight muscle tissue shortly after the onset of flight; an 80% decrease within 15 min of flight has been observed (Wegener et al., 1986). Fructose 2,6-bisphosphate is a potent activator of phosphofructokinases, and in vitro a decrease in fructose 2,6-bisphosphate concentration, corresponding to that observed in vivo, would reduce the activity of locust phosphofructokinase by 95% (Wegener et al., 1987a). Fructose 2,6-bisphosphate has therefore been attributed a role in sparing carbohydrate in sustained flight. It is not known whether this phenomenon is restricted to insects or whether it represents a general mechanism that is more clearly expressed in insect flight muscle than in other muscles that are capable of sustained exercise.

Physical Activity and Longevity

It is common knowledge that a certain amount of physical exercise is beneficial for developing and maintaining "fitness" of body functions in humans and animals alike. It is not known, however, whether the amount of exercise carried out during a lifetime would affect longevity. Exercise gives rise to an increase in metabolic rate, and there have been speculations that the metabolic rate is inversely related to life span. The problem can hardly be studied in humans. Experiments in insects have led to puzzling results and provoking hypotheses. Honey bees grow rather old when kept nonflying in the hive, whereas foraging greatly reduces their expectation of life (Neukirch, 1982). In houseflies (*Musca domestica*), in one series of experiments, to achieve different levels of activity, the wings were or were not excised from young flies. In other experiments, flies were singly confined to small bottles, where they could only walk, and compared to those kept in company in larger cages where flight was possible. "High activity flies" had shorter average and maximum life spans than "low activity flies" (for review, see Sohal & Allen, 1985). These effects could have been brought about by different, but not necessarily mutually exclusive, mechanisms. "High activity" or some parameter connected with it could have an immediate effect by overstraining some vital process, thus causing an increased risk of death (i.e., shortening the life span). On the other hand, high activity could have exerted a lasting, irreversible effect on life expectancy (i.e., accelerated aging). The "rate of living" theory of aging claims that a given species, under given environmental conditions, has a fixed metabolic potential (total energy expenditure per lifetime) and that the rate at which this energy is expended (i.e., the metabolic rate) would determine the actual duration of life. Support for this view comes from the observation that the rate at which the "age pigment" lipofuscin is deposited in some tissues of the fly (surprisingly, there is no lipofuscin in flight muscle) is correlated to the level of activity, and that the total amount of oxygen consumed per lifetime appears to be independent of the level of physical activity. However, Drosophila males that had been kept at a high reproductive activity (resulting in high mortality) during the first half of their life span acquired a lower mortality for the rest of their lives when no more females were provided, and their expectation of life was then indiscernible from controls that had been celibate throughout life. Hence, the reduced longevity at high reproductive activity would appear temporary and not caused by an acceleration of aging (Partridge & Andrews, 1985). Clearly, more experiments, combined with stringent control experiments, are necessary to evaluate the relationship between metabolic rate, life span, and other variables.

It is not known whether there is an effect of a high level of voluntary physical exercise on longevity in man. Elite marathon runners take up 4 l of O_2 per min during a race, and their training may cause an extra energy expenditure exceeding 40,000 kJ per week (Newsholme & Leech, 1983). Most endurance runners would agree that the time on the track counts twice with respect to the zest for life. It is trusted that this is not the case as far as life span is concerned.

Acknowledgments

Research of the author was supported by grants from the Deutsche Forschungsgemeinschaft, D-5300 Bonn.

References

Beenakkers, A.M.Th., Van der Horst, D.J., & Van Marrewijk, W.J.A. (1984). Insect flight muscle metabolism. *Insect Biochem.*, **14**, 243-260.

Herreid II, C.F., & Fourtner, C.R. (1981). *Locomotion and Energetics in Arthropods*. Plenum Press, New York.

Herreid II, C.F., & Full, R.J. (1984). Cockroaches on a treadmill: Aerobic running. *J. Insect Physiol.*, **30**, 395-403.

Kammer, A.E., & Heinrich, B. (1978). Insect flight metabolism. *Adv. Insect Physiol.,* **13**, 133-228.

Neukirch, A. (1982). Dependence of the life span of the honey bee (Apis mellifica) upon flight performance and energy consumption. *J. Comp. Physiol.,* **146**, 35-40.

Newsholme, E.A., & Leech, A.R. (1983). *Biochemistry for the medical sciences.* John Wiley and Sons, Chichester, New York.

Partridge, L., & Andrews, R. (1985). The effect of reproductive activity on the longevity of male Drosophila melanogaster is not caused by an acceleration of ageing. *J. Insect Physiol.,* **31**, 393-395.

Rowan, A.N., & Newsholme, E.A. (1979). Changes in the contents of nucleotides and intermediates of glycolysis and the citric acid cycle in flight muscle of the locust upon flight and their relationship to the control of the cycle. *Biochem. J.,* **178**, 209-216.

Sohal, R.S., & Allen, R.G. (1985). Relationship between metabolic rate, free radicals, differentiation and aging: A unified theory. In A.D. Woodhead, A.D. Blackett, & A. Hollaender (Eds.), *Molecular biology of aging.* Plenum, New York, 75-104.

Tucker, V.A. (1973). Aerial and terrestrial locomotion: A comparison of energetics. In L. Bolis, K. Schmidt-Nielsen, & S.H.P. Maddrell (Eds.), *Comparative physiology: Locomotion, respiration, transport, and blood.* North Holland Publ., Amsterdam, 63-76.

Wegener, G., Beinhauer, I., Klee, A., & Newsholme, E.A. (1987a). Properties of locust muscle 6-phosphofructokinase and their importance in the regulation of glycolytic flux during prolonged flight. *J. Comp. Physiol. B,* **57**, 315-326.

Wegener, G., Beinhauer, I., & Yonge, R. (1987b). Die Aktivierung der Glykolyse beim Insektenflug. *Verh. Dtsch. Zool. Ges.,* **80**, 230.

Wegener, G., Michel, R., & Newsholme, E.A. (1986). Fructose 2,6-bisphosphate as a signal for changing from sugar to lipid oxidation during flight in locusts. *FEBS Lett.,* **201**, 128-131.

Weis-Fogh, T. (1952). Fat combustion and metabolic rate of flying locusts (Schistocerca gregaria Forskål). *Phil. Trans. R. Soc.,* **B 237**, 1-36.

RESEARCH NOTES

Heparin-Induced Elevation of Plasma FFA and Exercise Metabolism in Dogs

Z. Brzezińska, D. Kruk, K. Nazar, H. Kaciuba-Uściłko, and S. Kozłowski

Department of Applied Physiology, Medical Research Centre, Polish Academy of Sciences, Warsaw, Poland

It has been demonstrated in few experimental studies that metabolic responses to physical effort can be largely modified by dietary modifications (Jansson & Kaijser, 1982; Maughan et al., 1978; Nazar, 1981; Rennie & Johnson, 1974). Rennie et al. (1976) demonstrated that glycogen utilization in contracting red skeletal muscles and in the liver is significantly slower in rats exercising after a fat meal followed by heparin injection than in control animals on a standard diet. The aim of this work was to elucidate an influence of elevated plasma FFA concentration, due to intravascular lipolysis, on work performance and exercise metabolism.

Material and Methods

The experiments were carried out on 10 male mongrel dogs exercising until exhaustion (a) after 20 to 22 h fasting (control experiments-C) or (b) 4 h after ingestion of 100 ml of soya bean oil followed by iv injection of heparin given immediately before starting the run (FFA experiments). The slope of the treadmill was 21% and its speed varied from 4.2 to 5.8 km • h^{-1}, depending on the individual capacity of each dog. During all exercise tests, oxygen uptake (VO_2), rectal temperature (T_{re}), and heart rate (HR) were recorded, and each 30 min venous blood samples were taken for measurements of blood glucose (BG) and lactate (LA) concentrations by enzymatic methods (Germed, GDR), plasma FFA level by the enzymatic method of Shimazu et al. (1979), and glycerol and triacylglycerol (TG) concentrations by enzymatic methods, using kits purchased from Boehringer (Mannheim, FRG). Needle bioptic samples of vastus lateralis were obtained at the same time from points under local anesthesia for determinations of glycogen, free glucose, hexose phosphates, pyruvate (PA), LA, creatine phosphate (CrP), creatine (Cr), ATP, ADP, and AMP. Muscle samples were freeze-dried and powdered.

Results

Exercise duration was shortened in 50% of dogs with elevated FFA. Exercise-induced increases in HR and T_{re} were higher in FFA than in C experiments. It was accompanied

Table 1 Changes in Muscle ATP, ADP, AMP, CrP, and Cr Contents as Well as in ATP/ADP Molar Ratio During Control and FFA Experiments in Dogs

	Control experiments				FFA experiments		
	0	30 min	75 min	91 min	0	30 min	75 min
Muscle ATP (μmol · g^{-1})	23.3 ± 0.63	22.4 ± 0.65	22.0 ± 0.64	22.0 ± 0.84	22.5 ± 0.68	21.0 ± 0.87	19.9 ± 1.06
Muscle ADP (μmol · g^{-1})	3.43 ± 0.24	3.80 ± 0.24	4.29 ± 0.29	4.38 ± 0.25	3.54 ± 0.30	4.56 ± 0.31*	5.14 ± 0.49*
Muscle ATP/ADP molar ratio	7.18 ± 0.53	6.15 ± 0.45	5.30 ± 0.52	5.14 ± 0.53	6.85 ± 0.61	4.89 ± 0.47	4.49 ± 0.62
Muscle AMP (μmol · g^{-1})	0.19 ± 0.02	0.25 ± 0.05	0.30 ± 0.06	0.28 ± 0.04	0.23 ± 0.03	0.28 ± 0.04	0.33 ± 0.13
Muscle CrP (μmol · g^{-1})	75.8 ± 2.4	56.5 ± 2.4	50.2 ± 1.9	46.2 ± 2.8	76.4 ± 2.7	55.0 ± 3.7	40.7 ± 2.8
Muscle Cr (μmol · g^{-1})	40.7 ± 2.0	58.2 ± 3.4	67.8 ± 2.8	70.7 ± 3.1	39.4 ± 1.5	60.9 ± 2.9**	82.2 ± 3.8**

Note. Values are means ± *SE*. Significant differences between control and FFA experiments are indicated by asterisks: *$p < .05$; **$p < .01$.

by lowered RQ and a tendency toward an enhanced $\dot{V}O_2$. Concentrations of the plasma FFA, glycerol, and TG were markedly higher in FFA experiments than in C without any significant differences in BG and LA levels. In dogs with elevated plasma FFA, the exercise-induced muscle glycogen depletion was reduced, muscle free glucose and hexose phosphate contents were elevated, while PA and LA contents were only slightly lower than in C experiments. Exercise-induced decreases in muscle CrP and ATP contents as well as in the ATP/ADP molar ratio were more pronounced in FFA than in C experiments (Table 1).

Conclusion

The study demonstrated that increased availability of FFA for working muscles exerts an inhibitory effect on both glycogen and glucose metabolism. In spite of the carbohydrate sparing effect of FFA, their excess does not improve work performance at moderate intensity, most probably because of enhanced energy expenditure, oxygen demand, and more pronounced hyperthermia.

Acknowledgments

This work was supported by the Polish Central Programme for Basic Research 06-02-III.2.1.

References

Jansson, E., & Kaijser, L. (1982). Effect of diet on the utilization of blood-borne and intramuscular substrates during exercise in man. *Acta Physiol. Scand.*, **115**, 19-30.

Maughan, R.J., Williams, C., Campbell, D.M., & Hepburn, D. (1978). Fat and carbohydrate metabolism during low intensity exercise: Effects of the availability of muscle glycogen. *Eur. J. Appl. Physiol.*, **39**, 7-16.

Nazar, K. (1981). Glucostatic control of hormonal response to physical exercise in men. In J. Poortmans & G. Niset (Eds.), *Biochemistry of exercise IV*. University Park Press, Baltimore, 188-196.

Rennie, M.J., & Johnson, R.H. (1974). Effect of an exercise–diet program on metabolic changes with exercise in runners. *J. Appl. Physiol.*, **37**, 821-825.

Rennie, M.J., Winder, W.W., & Holloszy, J.O. (1976). A sparing effect of increased free fatty acids on muscle glycogen content in exercising rat. *Biochem. J.*, **156**, 647-655.

Shimazu, S., Inoue, K., Tani, Y., & Yamada, H. (1979). Enzymatic microdetermination of serum free fatty acids. *Analyt. Biochem.*, **98**, 341-345.

Blood Platelet Superoxide Dismutase Activity and Malonyldialdehyde Concentrations in Healthy Men Following Submaximal Physical Exercise

A. Buczyński, J. Błaszczyk, and J. Kędziora

Department of Physiology, Institute of Fundamental Sciences, Military School of Medicine, Łódź, Poland

Physical exercise, as one of numerous factors stimulating cellular oxidative metabolism, may be expected to increase free oxygen radical generation responsible for lipid peroxidation. Therefore, we decided to determine the effect of physical exercise on blood platelet superoxide (SOD-1) activity and malonyldialdehyde (MDA) concentration in healthy men.

Material and Methods

Our investigations were performed with 11 healthy men, aged 20 to 23 years, always at the same time of the day. During 3 weeks preceding the studies the subjects were not given any compounds affecting blood platelet function. All of them were subjected to submaximal physical exercise on bicycle ergometer at a load of 2 W/kg of body weight for 15 minutes. Before and after exercise blood samples, withdrawn from the cubital vein, were mixed in polyethylene tubes with 1% EDTA in 0.14 M NaCl solution at a ratio of 1:9. Blood platelets were isolated by means of fractioned centrifugation (Aharony et al., 1982; Holmsen, 1980). The obtained blood platelet suspension contained less than 0.01% of other blood cells. Blood platelet SOD-1 activity was determined according to Misra and Fridovich (Misra & Fridovich, 1972) with our own modification, while MDA concentrations were assayed according to Placer et al. (1966). Statistical analysis was performed with paired Student's t test. In relation to the resting values, physical exercise induced a significant rise in blood platelet SOD-1 activity and a decrease in blood platelet MDA concentration.

Discussion

Free oxygen radicals have particular affinity to cell membranes and they induce membrane lipid peroxidation, leading to membrane damage and changes in its biological properties (Michael et al., 1985). Cellular antioxidant system, including SOD-1, glutathione peroxidase and catalase, protects cells from toxic action of free oxygen radicals. Since physical exercise stimulates cellular oxidative metabolism, an increased free oxygen radical generation and lipid peroxidation may be expected. It has been reported that in some persons physical exercise induces lipid peroxidation responsible for augmented aggregation of blood platelets (Ross, 1983; Scheale & Müller, 1978), although Mathis et al. (1981) have not confirmed these findings. Results of our studies seem to indicate that physical exercise limits lipid peroxidation, thereby reducing blood platelet activation.

References

Aharony, D., Smith, J.B., & Silver, M.J. (1982). Regulation of arachidonate induced platelet aggregation by the lipooxygenase product 12 hydroxyeicosatetrenosic acid. *Biochim. Biophys. Acta*, **718**, 193-197.

Holmsen, H. (1980). Energy metabolism of platelet responses. *Vox Sang*,. **40**, 1-7.

Mathis, C.P., Wohl, H., Wallack, S.R., & Engler, R.I. (1981). Lack of release of platelet factor 4 during exercise-induced myocardial ischemia. *N.E.J. Med*,. **309**, 1275-1279.

Brown, M.S., & Goldstein, J.L. (1985). How LDL receptors influence cholesterol and atherosclerosis. *Scientific American*, **10**, 56-60.

Misra, H.P., & Fridovich, J. (1972). The role of superoxide anion in the autooxidation of epinephrine and a simple assay superoxide dismutase. *J. Biol. Chem*,. **247**, 3170-3173.

Placer, Z., Cushman, L., & Jonson, B. (1966). Estimation of product of lipid peroxidation malonyldialdehyde in biochemical systems. *Anal. Bioch*,. **16**, 359-364.

Ross, R. (1983). Platelets and atherosclerosis. *Arzneimittel Forschung*, **33**, 1399-1401.

Scheale, K., & Müller, K.M. (1978). Acute cardiac death caused by an increase of platelet aggregation during and after maximal physical stress. In T. Libich & A. Venerando (Eds.), *Sports cardiology*. Bologna, 203-211.

Gamma–Glutamyltransferase and Physical Exercise

H. Ohno, Y. Sato, T. Yahata, A. Kuroshima, K. Yamamura, and N. Taniguchi

Asahikawa Medical College, Asahikawa; Research Center of Health, Physical Fitness and Sports, Nagoya University, Nagoya; and Osaka University Medical School, Osaka, Japan

It has been shown that strenuous exercise decreases liver glutathione level and that physically trained rats eliminate drugs at a faster rate. γ-Glutamyltransferase (γGT), which is present in large amounts in the microsomal fraction, catalyzes the initial step in the breakdown of the glutathione in tissue. However, there are very few reports as to the effect of physical exercise on γGT. In addition, it is γGT activity that has been traditionally measured, but not the mass of the protein of which the enzyme is mainly composed; however, such measurement may not reflect the true amount of the enzyme protein, due to the presence or absence of cofactors, activators, and inhibitors. Hereupon, we examined the effect of physical exercise on both the activity and concentration of γGT in men and rats.

In experiments with men, the effects of physical training on plasma activity and concentration of γGT were investigated with 7 previously sedentary healthy males students, aged 18 to 19 years. The training protocol consisted of running over 5 km, 6 times/week for 10 weeks. An enzyme-linked immunosorbent assay (ELISA) for human plasma immunoreactive γGT was done as previously described (Taniguchi et al., 1985). One unit of γGT was defined as 1 μmol of p-nitrophenol released per minute at 30 °C. The subjects' mean maximal oxygen uptake ($\dot{V}O_2$max) and 12-minute field performance increased significantly after training, from 43.5 and 2683 to 48.1 ml $\cdot$ kg^{-1} $\cdot$ min^{-1} and 2931 m, respectively, indicating improvement in aerobic capacity.

After training, the resting plasma γGT concentration ($\pm SE$) decreased markedly from 20.4 (± 2.3) to 10.1 μg $\cdot$ ml^{-1} (± 0.9), whereas the γGT activity did not change substantially. The training did not affect the response to the $\dot{V}O_2$max test of either concentration or activity of γGT.

In experiments on rats, 15 male Wistar strain rats (EX, 9 wk old), with an average weight of 220 g, were exercised by swimming until exhausted with a weight equal to 3% of their body weight in water at 34 to 36 °C. Ten 4-week, cold-acclimated (5 °C) male rats (CA, 11 wk old) weighing approximately 246 g and 6 cold-adapted rats (CG, 11 wk old), weighing 219 g, reared in cold for 40 successive generations were also studied. Eleven warm-adapted male rats (11 wk old, 282 g) served as controls. Microsomal γGT was studied in liver cell fractions of all rats. Tissue preparations and an ELISA for rat immunoreactive γGT were made according to the method of Taniguchi et al. (1983). In vivo and in vitro permeabilities for both γGT activity and content were calculated by the following formulas of Toncsev and Frenkl (1984):

$$\text{In vivo permeability (\%)} = \frac{\text{extramicrosomal fraction} \times 100}{\text{extramicrosomal fraction} + \text{microsomal fraction}}$$

and

$$\text{in vitro permeability (\%)} = \frac{\text{hyposmotic condition}}{\text{isosmotic condition}} \times 100$$

γGT in the microsomal fraction was observed in the presence of 0.2% Triton X-100 dissolved in isotonic, 0.25 M sucrose. In the experiments on the in vitro release of γGT, 1.0 ml of pellet containing intact microsomes was incubated at 37 °C in isotonic sucrose or distilled water at pH 7.4 for 1 hour (for details see Toncsev & Frenkl, 1984).

In both extramicrosomal and microsomal fractions, protein contents in EX decreased significantly, but in CA and CG they increased. γGT activities elevated significantly in the extramicrosomal fraction of EX and in the microsomal fraction of CA and CG. γGT contents appeared to increase only in the microsomal fraction of CG. In vivo permeability of γGT activity was greatly enhanced on EX but reduced on CA and CG, while the in vitro permeability did not vary significantly. On the other hand, in vivo permeability of γGT content changed significantly only on EX. In vitro permeability of γGT content seemed to decrease on CA and CG.

The present study may lead to the following conclusions: (a) Plasma γGT concentration in humans is useful as an index of extent of physical training. (b) Immunoreactive γGT does not always correlate with the enzyme activity. (c) Acute exercise increases the permeability of the microsomal membrane of rat liver. (d) Cold adaptation stabilizes the membrane of the liver microsomes.

References

Taniguchi, N., Iizuka, S., Zhe, Z.N., House, S., Yokosawa, N., Ono, M., Kinoshita, K., Makita, A., & Sekiya, C. (1985). Measurement of human serum immunoreactive γ-glutamyl transpeptidase in patients with malignant tumors using enzyme-linked immunosorbent assay. *Cancer Res.*, **45**, 5835-5839.

Taniguchi, N., Yokosawa, N., Iizuka, S., Sako, F., Tsukada, Y., Satoh, M., & Dempo, K. (1983). γ-Glutamyl transpeptidase of rat liver and hepatoma tissues: an enzyme immunoassay and immunostaining studies. *Ann. N.Y. Acad. Sci.*, **417**, 203-212.

Toncsev, H. & Frenkl, R. (1984). Studies on the lysosomal enzyme system of the liver in rats undergoing swimming training. *Int. J. Sports Med.*, **5**, 152-155.

Physiological Responses to Physical Exercise at the Anaerobic Threshold Level

T. Boraczyński and R. Zdanowicz

Department of Physiology, Academy of Physical Education, Warsaw, Poland

Eight novice middle-distance runners aged 17.3 $\pm$ 0.9 years performed 30-min treadmill exercise at a speed equal to the individual anaerobic threshold ($V_2 = AT_{ind}$) and at that speed lowered by 1 km $\cdot$ h^{-1} ($V_1 < AT_{ind}$). At the speed below AT_{ind} exercise was executed under functional equilibrium with only slight increases in blood lactate concentration (LA) from 2.26 $\pm$ 0.56 to 2.45 $\pm$ 0.18 mmol $\cdot$ L^{-1}. During running at the speed equal to AT_{ind} an initial increase of blood LA concentration was followed by its stabilization at the average level of 5.3 mmol $\cdot$ L^{-1}. It was accompanied by a gradual decrease of blood HCO_3 and pCO_2 and an increase of pulmonary ventilation, while blood pH remained at the resting level throughout the exercise. During both types of exercise, below and at AT_{ind}, a linear increase of heart rate was observed. The results have shown that the individual anaerobic threshold, determined in the laboratory progressive-speed exercise, may be used as a determinant of the intensity of endurance exercise of up to 30-min duration.

The Interrelationship Between Aerobic and Anaerobic Performance in Athletes

A. Jaskólski, A. Jaskólska, and J. Krawczak

Department of Physiology, College of Physical Education, Poznań Faculty of Physiology Education, Gorzów Wlkp., Poland

The aim of this study was to evaluate interrelationships between indices of aerobic and anaerobic capacity in middle-distance runners. Six healthy middle-distance runners aged 21.2 ± 1.8 years with body weight of 68.8 ± 1.96 kg were examined. Aerobic power and total work performed during incremental tests on cycloergometer were determined. To estimate anaerobic power and capacity, the Wingate test on the Monark ergometer was performed. The following indices of anaerobic performance were calculated: peak power (PP), mean power (MP), and power decrease (PD). Correlation coefficients were calculated to assess the relationships between aerobic and anaerobic performance. The results are summarized in Tables 1 and 2. This study showed high positive correlations between aerobic capacity of middle-distance runners and indices of anaerobic performance (i.e., the peak and mean power attained during the Wingate test).

Table 1   Indices of Aerobic and Anaerobic Performance in the Subjects Examined

Variable	$\bar{X}$	±	SD
Peak power (W)	713.15		79.21
(W · kg BW^{-1})	10.39		1.02
Mean power (W)	583.96		55.85
(W · kg BW^{-1})	8.59		0.69
Power decrease (W · s^{-1})	9.68		1.36
$\dot{V}O_2$max (L · min^{-1})	4.39		0.33
(ml · kg^{-1} · min^{-1})	63.97		3.49
Total work (kJ)	148.38		18.67
(kJ · kg BW^{-1})	2.16		0.22

Note. N = 6.

Table 2   Correlation Matrix for Aerobic and Anaerobic Performance

Variables	1	2	3	4
1 Peak power (BW)				
2 Mean power (BW)	0.936**			
3 Power decrease	0.427	0.168		
4 $\dot{V}O_2$max (BW)	0.945**	0.867*	0.553	
5 Total work (BW)	0.773	0.669	0.716	0.916*

*$p < .05$. **$p < .01$.

Lactic Acid Removal, Changes in Acid–Base Balance and Kinetics of Growth Hormone at Rest and During Controlled Recovery Exercise

B. Opaszowski, J. Łukaszewska, M. Sienicka, and S. Furdal

Department of Physiology, Academy of Physical Educátion and Institute of Sport, Warsaw, Poland

The purpose of this study was to compare lactic acid removal, changes in acid–base balance, and growth hormone levels during passive and active recovery from supramaximal exercise. Five healthy men (23-25 years) volunteered for this study. Their maximal oxygen uptake ($\dot{V}O_2$max) was 51 to 61 ml • kg^{-1} • min^{-1}. On the first day (Test I) the subjects ran three times on the treadmill at a speed which led to exhaustion within 60 s with rest periods of 4 min between the runs. In the recovery period (40 min) the subjects rested in sitting position. On the 2nd day (Test II) after the same supramaximal intermittent exercise the subjects ran at a speed representing 60% of their $\dot{V}O_2$max for 30 min. On the 3rd day (Test III), the subjects ran at 60% $\dot{V}O_2$max for 30 min. Capillary blood samples were taken before exercise, after the supramaximal intermittent exercise, and at the 5th, 10th, 20th, 30th, and 40th min of the passive or active recovery periods. Growth hormone (GH), lactic acid (LA), pH, HCO$_3$, and pCO$_2$ levels in the plasma were determined. GH levels in Test I were higher than those in Test II or III. The estimations of blood LA, pH, HCO$_3$, and pCO$_2$ showed that active recovery is more effective than passive recovery. There were linear correlations between GH levels and LA ($r = .866$), pH ($r = .678$), HCO$_3$ ($r = .683$), and pCO$_2$ ($r = -.579$). The results suggest that an increase in blood LA and/or changes in acid–base balance stimulate GH release.

Working Ability and Exercise Metabolism in Dogs Deprived of Food for One Week

K. Nazar, Z. Brzezińska, J. Langfort, B. Kruk, I. Falęcka-Wieczorek, W. Pilis, and H. Kaciuba-Uściłko

Department of Applied Physiology, Medical Research Centre, Polish Academy of Sciences, Warsaw, Poland

Metabolic responses to treadmill exercise of moderate (max duration approximately 50 min) and high (max duration approximately 15 min) intensities were compared in male mongrel dogs before and after 1 week of fasting. Food deprivation caused a decrease in body weight by approximately 2.1 kg (i.e., 11.2% of the initial body mass), a decrease in resting HR, and a marked increase in the plasma FFA concentration without any significant changes in blood glucose (BG), glycerol, and lactate (LA) levels. Glycogen content in skeletal muscles (vastus lateralis) was reduced by 50%, which was accompanied by diminished glucose and hexose phosphate contents and an increase in pyruvate and LA contents. Ability to perform the moderate (8 dogs) and heavy (7 dogs) exercise was not affected. Blood FFA, glycerol, glucose, and LA responses to both kinds of exercise did not differ before and after food deprivation. The exercise-induced muscle glycogen breakdown was smaller in fasted than in control animals; however, the postexercise values of glycogen were lower in the former. After the exercise of high intensity, muscle contents of glucose, hexose phosphates, and LA were lower in fasting dogs while during the effort of moderate intensity these differences were insignificant. Fasting did not induce any pronounced changes in muscle adenine nucleotide and creatine phosphate responses to exercise. It is concluded that in dogs performance of aerobic exercises, even of heavy intensity, is not impaired by deprivation of food for several days in spite of markedly diminished body carbohydrate reserves.

Serum Glycogenolytic Activity in Exercising Rats Measured in Vitro

T. Torlińska and L. Torliński

Department of Physiology and Department of Medical Biochemistry, Karol Marcinkowski Medical Academy of Poznań, Poland

In the first part of this study the effect of exercise on some blood constituents and tissue glycogen concentrations was examined in rats swimming for 30 min in tepid water (32 °C). The exercise resulted in a decrease in glycogen content in the liver (by 60%) and skeletal muscle (by 35%), an increase in serum glucose, lactate, and FFA levels (by 51%, 25%, and 59%, respectively) as well as in an increase in plasma glucagon and corticosterone concentrations (by 18% and 40%). Adrenaline and noradrenaline contents in the adrenals were decreased by 14% and 38%, respectively. In the second part of this study serum glycogenolytic activity (SGA) in exercising rats was determined in vitro. For this purpose 500 mg of fresh liver slices taken from control (sedentary) rats were incubated at 37 °C with 0.5 ml of the exercising rat serum diluted in 9.5 ml of a solution containing 125 mM NaCl, 6 mM KCl, 1 mM $CaCl_2$, 1.2 mM $MgSO_4$, 1 mM NaH_2PO_4, 5 mM $NaHCO_3$, and 2 mM sodium pyruvate with pH 7.4. SGA was expressed as micromoles of glucose released by factors present in 0.5 ml of the tested serum per g w.w. of liver slices per 1 hour. SGA of exercising rats was increased by 71% as compared with that of controls. Regitine (alpha adrenergic blocker) and insulin added in vitro produced a fall in SGA which was more pronounced than that found following propranolol and insulin. These results indicate that glycogenolysis in the rat liver is predominantly stimulated by alpha–adrenergic receptor system.

Signs of Fatigue During Exercise on the Kayak Ergometer

I. Wojcieszak, E. Michael, G. Lutosławska, and J. Wojczuk

Department of Physiology and Biochemistry, Institute of Sport, Warsaw, Poland and Department of Education, University of California, Santa Barbara, USA

The purpose of this study was to recognize causes of fatigue occurring in kayakers during paddling a distance of 1000 m. The dependence of oxygen uptake, oxygen debt, EMG, lactic acid (LA), and ammonia blood concentrations on duration of the effort was studied. The subjects were 11 male kayakers. A specific test for kayakers (4 min) was applied using a kayak ergometer. In successive studies the exercise was interrupted after 1, 2, 3, and 4 min. During each exercise test the power and amount of work performed was determined and $\dot{V}O_2$ was measured during exercise and during 10 minutes of the recovery period. LA concentration was determined 1, 4, 8, 15, and 30 min after termination of the effort. Venous blood ammonia was tested before and immediately after exercise. It was found that the decline in power output during the specific test was accompanied by a progressive increase in the concentration of blood LA and ammonia as well as by an increase in $\dot{V}O_2$ and oxygen debt. $\dot{V}O_2$ per unit of work (kJ) increased and the amount of LA per unit of power declined with duration of exercise. It seems that fatigue developing during 4 min of exercise on a kayak ergometer is caused by the factors connected with acidosis of the upper extremity muscles, resulting in reduction of the muscle ability to perform work.

Part III
Energy Metabolism and Its Control

Nutritional Individuality and Physical Performance in Different Periods of Life

J. Pařizková

Research Institute for Physical Education, Charles University, Prague, Czechoslovakia

Nutrition is one of the closest links of an organism with its environment. Especially during certain periods of development such as suckling, weaning, or puberty, nutritional manipulations, in both positive and negative ways, can influence the organism profoundly, sometimes with delayed effects.

Physical activity and exercise are the most important variables increasing energy output above the basal level. Recommended allowances were elaborated in most industrially developed countries. Nevertheless, such recommendations, for example, the last one from the World Health Organization (Geneva, 1985) can serve only as general guidelines, since marked interindividual differences exist in various population groups classified according to age, sex, physical work loads, and so forth. "Nutritional individuality" develops from the very beginning of life (Widdowson, 1962) and therefore, under similar conditions and even in individuals with very closely related characteristics, food is absorbed and utilized according to varying metabolic stereotypes. This variability is explained by both genetic and constitutional factors, as well as by some adaptive processes occurring during life; the adaptation to various energy outputs according to various work loads is considered as one of the most important.

Nutrition and Physical Activity in Experimental Animals

The adaptive processes caused by various diets and/or exercise can have a particularly immediate impact during certain developmental periods such as that of nutritional dependence on breast milk or puberty. Experimental animals (male rats) kept in nests of different sizes (more than 12 or fewer than 6 rats per cage) showed, after weaning, various levels of spontaneous physical activity as assessed in rotation wheels. Males from large nests, those having less mother's milk, showed significantly higher spontaneous activity from the 60th day of life until the end of the experiment (85 days) as compared to males from small nests. Females in general had a higher level of motor activity in comparison with males of comparable age; no additional effect of decreased milk intake was observed. Epididymal fat pads were significantly lighter and the percentage of the total body fat was lower in males from large nests. Number of offspring fed by one mother influenced later in life some metabolic variables in both males and females. Total lipid content, lipogenesis, and synthesis of fatty acids in the small intestine were significantly increased in animals of both sexes from large nests. The content of fatty acids in the liver as well as synthesis of cholesterol in the carcass were significantly higher in both males and females from large nests (Pařizková, 1978a; Pařizková & Petrásek, 1979; Pařizková et al., 1979).

There exist other models of reduced nutrition early in life, for example, a diet with only 10% of proteins given to females during lactation, and then with only 5% of proteins up to the 7th week of the offspring's life (temporary protein-energy malnutrition—PEM). Such a diet causes a significantly smaller body weight increase and reduced fatness, resulting again in significantly increased levels of spontaneous physical activity in male offspring. In this experiment significantly increased contents of total lipids along with reduced liposynthesis in the liver were also found. These findings may be explained by an increased lipid mobilization with simultaneously reduced lipid synthesis due to the increased physical activity and energy output. Fatty acid levels and the rate of their synthesis in the liver, cholesterol concentration, and its synthesis in the liver and cholesterolemia did not differ significantly (Pařizková et al., 1979, 1980).

Nutritional manipulations early in life can lead to a higher level of spontaneous physical activity along with a changed food intake, body weight, and certain indices of lipid metabolism. On the other hand, it is of interest that increased physical activity of female rats during pregnancy resulted in significant changes in the offspring. In this experiment pregnant rats were exercised for 1 hour per day on a treadmill, and the microstructure of the heart was examined in male offspring at the age of 100 days of postnatal life. The offspring of exercised mothers had larger hearts with significantly increased density of muscle fibers and capillaries, elevated capillary to fibre ratio, shorter diffusion distance (Pařizková, 1978b) and showed some differences in lipid metabolism (Pařizková & Petrásek, 1979). When exercise of the offspring was continued, both male and female physically active rats born from exercised mothers had the highest densities of fibers and capillaries in the heart, and shortest diffusion distances, whereas the control inactive offspring of the control sedentary mothers had the lowest of these variables (Figures 1 and 2). Both the pre- and postnatal work loads cause changes in the microstructure of the heart which are considered favorable for physical work capacity.

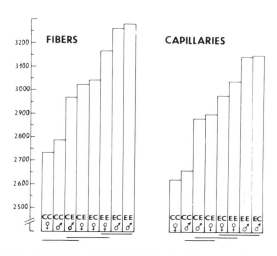

Figure 1. Multiple range test of the number of fibers and capillaries per square mm in the heart of the rats subjected to different physical activity regimes during prenatal and postnatal ontogenesis. Each pair of groups underlined at least by one line does not differ significantly. *Note.* CC = control offspring of control mothers, CE = exercised offspring of control mothers, EC = control offspring of exercised mothers, EE = exercised offspring of exercised mothers.

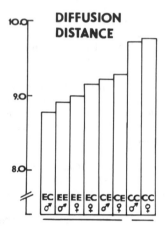

Figure 2. Multiple range test of the diffusion distance D/2 in the heart of the rats subjected to different physical activity regimes during prenatal and postnatal ontogenesis. See note to Figure 1. From Pǎrizková (1979).

Treadmill exercise (1-4 hours per day) during postnatal development decreased the total and epididymal fat pad weights, and reduced the degree of cardiac lesions induced by application of isoprenaline and followed by the ^{203}HgCl injection. This was demonstrated by a decreased CPM (counts per minute) and decreased accumulation index (relating CPM • body weight^{-1} to CPM • g heart weight^{-1}) (Faltová et al., 1983, 1985). The adaptation to prolonged exercise was associated with an increased resistance of myocardium to necrogenic effect of isoprenaline as shown previously (Parizková & Faltova, 1970).

Rats with early protein energy malnutrition (PEM) exercising in the rotation wheels had smaller cardiac lesions after isoprenaline at the age of 105 days then sedentary PEM animals and control exercising animals. The worst in this respect were the ad libitum fed animals (Figure 3) without any exercise (Pařizková et al., 1982).

Nutritional and physical activity changes early in life can result in modifications of somatic development, body composition, and metabolic and motor activity development which become apparent only later in life. One could speculate whether situations analogous to those observed in the above mentioned experimental models can be found in human subjects. There has been some evidence on the delayed consequences of early malnutrition and/or early motor stimulation for later human behavior and body development (Brozek & Schürch, 1984; Dobbing, 1984; Koch, 1976).

Studies With Human Subjects

The data concerning food intake in individual age categories and functional capacity, as characterized by the oxygen uptake during maximal work load, showed the corresponding trends: During the period of somatic growth both the energy intake per kg of body weight (kJ • kg^{-1}) and aerobic power (ml • kg^{-1} • min^{-1}) are the highest, and decrease later with increasing age (Pařizková, 1985a, 1986). This indicates the highest energy turnover and performance capacity of the cardiorespiratory system during the stages of most rapid growth and development with decreasing values in the middle and advanced age as related both to total and lean body mass (Figures 4 and 5).

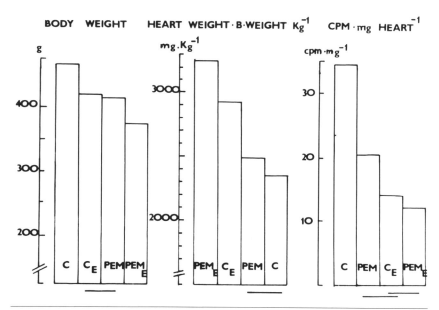

Figure 3. Multiple range test of body weight, relative heart weight, and the degree of cardiac lesion after the application of isoprenaline as characterized by counts per minute (CPM). From Pǎrizková et al. (1982).

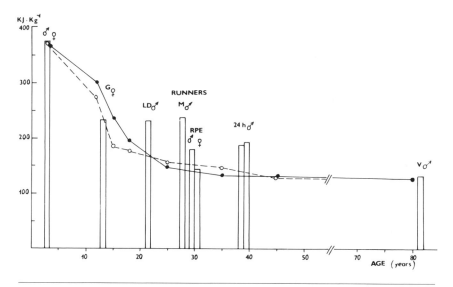

Figure 4. Daily energy intake per kg of body weight in normal population (-•-•- males; -o--o- females) and athletes. *Note.* first column = preschool children, G = girl gymnasts, LD = long distance, M = marathon runners, RPE = participants of recreation physical education (men and women), 24h = runners for 24 hours, V = old men.

108 Pařizková

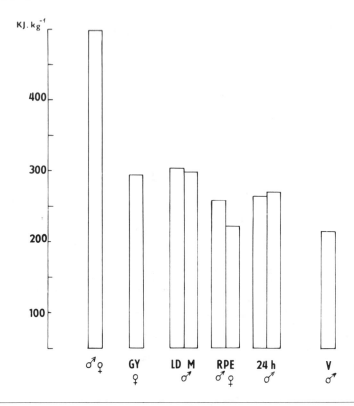

KJ. kg⁻¹

400

300

200

100

♂♀   GY   LD M   RPE   24 h   V
       ♀   ♂   ♂♀   ♂   ♂

Figure 5. Daily energy intake related to lean body mass in different groups of subjects. See note to Figure 4.

Long term sport activity requires, in certain disciplines, an increase in food intake. Therefore recommended dietary allowances (RDA) for groups of specialized athletes were elaborated (Hejda et al., 1978) according to differently increased or reduced energy needs. Figure 4 shows mean values of energy intake per kg of body weight in groups of children and athletes of different age and specialization as compared to the trends found in untrained population groups. As demonstrated in Figure 4 no differences in the energy intake per kg of body weight were found in preschool children (Pařizková et al., 1986) regardless of the level of their spontaneous physical activity. Girl gymnasts (12-14 years of age) who were preselected for national championships and who are often assumed to have a too low energy intake remained also within the range of the normal population. Moreover, when their weight and proportionality were plotted against the national growth grids, they were always within the range of standard values.

Nevertheless, there was found a wide variation in the individual energy intake ($V_{\bar{x}} = 14$-20). Groups of long distance runners and marathon runners had higher energy intake as compared to the normal untrained population, but they did not achieve RDA values based on the theoretically estimated energy output during training and competition (Pařizková, 1987). Again, a wide variation in energy intake was found between individuals in spite of very similar somatic development—height, weight, lean body mass, as well as the conditions of training and competition. The same applied to the intake of individual components of food—protein, fat, carbohydrates, minerals, and vitamins (Pařizková, 1985b). Similar variability of energy intake as related to body weight was found in other groups of athletes: A practically identical regime of exercise did not diminish the inter-individual variability. This seems to indicate that there exist apparently endogenic factors that influence the energy output, and therefore also the energy needs that are more important than the physical activity level.

Comparisons of groups of recreationally exercising subjects showed identical values of energy intake for women (Figure 4), and increased values for men as compared to the normal population. The changes in body composition in women were greater (i.e., their body fat was lower than in the control inactive population) than in men who showed more-over a less strict nutritional regime (lower frequency of meals per day, relatively bigger meals in the evening than during the day, etc.). Again, the variability among individuals was large; there were no relationships between energy intake to body weight, body composition, aerobic power, level of blood cholesterol, etc. (Pařizková et al., 1985a). However, it is necessary to consider that these individuals were characterized by a normal range of energy intake (i.e., obese or very lean subjects were excluded). Finally, the values of energy intake for men who lived rather long (until 81 years) corresponded well to normal population trends (Pařizková, 1983). The same applies to the intake of protein, fat, and carbohydrates (Figures 6-8).

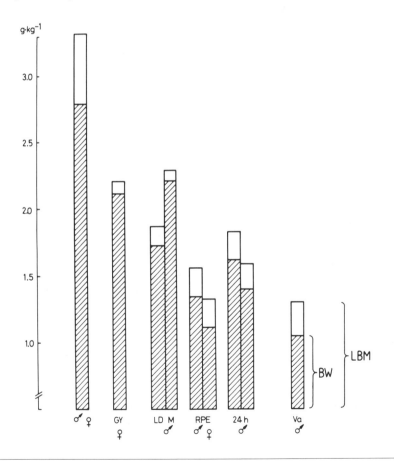

Figure 6. Daily protein intake per kg of body weight and/or lean body mass in different groups of subjects. See note to Figure 4.

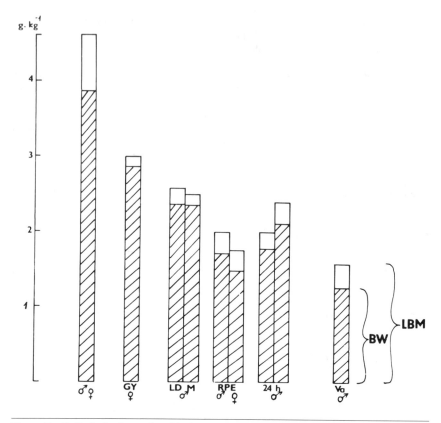

Figure 7. Daily fat intake per kg of body weight and/or lean body mass in different groups of subjects. See note to Figure 4.

The large range of interindividual variability was also confirmed in the exceptional case of men training regularly for the 24-hour run. The measurements of mean energy intake and some main components of food ingested during three days prior to and on the day of the 24-hour run and four days afterwards showed once more a wide variety of values (Table 1). The mean age of these men was 38.55 years, their body mass index (BMI) was 21.9 and the average distance run during 24 hours was 176.5 km. The latter did not correlate with the energy intake, which also failed to relate to the aerobic power, or to any biochemical variables measured such as enzyme activities in skeletal muscle (quadriceps femoris muscle biopsies—citrate-synthetase, lactate dehydrogenase, hydroxyacyl-CoA-dehydrogenase) and the proportion of fast- and slow-twitch muscle fibers. Obviously, on the basis of up-to-date knowledge it is still difficult to explain the mechanisms underlying the variability of energy needs; it seems that individuals can get along even during very similar and demanding work loads with quite different energy and food component intakes achieving very similar levels of performance (Pařizková, 1987).

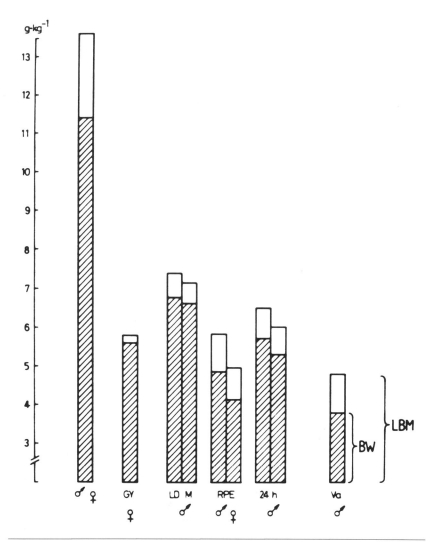

Figure 8. Daily carbohydrate intake per kg body weight and/or lean body mass in different groups of subjects. See note to Figure 4.

Conclusions

The above mentioned data seem to indicate that in addition to genetic factors and adaptational processes during postnatal life it is necessary to consider the impact of both energy intake and output determined mainly by diet and physical activity very early in life (i.e.,

Table 1   Food Intake in Men Performing 24-Hour Run

		3 days before the run	Breakfast before the run	24-hour run	4 days after the run
Energy (MJ)	$\bar{X}$	12.68	5.33	13.05	14.83
	SD	6.52	1.84	8.11	4.48
Proteins (g)					
total	$\bar{X}$	108.8	33.7	94.5	121.9
	SD	59.1	19.9	49.9	44.1
animal	$\bar{X}$	70.9	18.6	53.4	75.0
	SD	43.1	17.5	28.1	31.7
plant	$\bar{X}$	37.9	15.1	41.0	46.9
	SD	21.1	8.4	22.4	22.5
Fats (g)					
total	$\bar{X}$	119.4	68.1	141.6	144.5
	SD	66.6	40.7	96.8	67.6
animal	$\bar{X}$	91.4	34.6	90.2	95.1
	SD	57.4	45.6	40.3	43.4
plant	$\bar{X}$	28.0	33.5	51.3	49.5
	SD	27.6	37.8	64.4	42.8
Carbohydrates (g)	$\bar{X}$	384.5	134.8	358.1	461.4
	SD	195.4	33.9	247.3	191.9
Minerals (mg)					
Ca	$\bar{X}$	938	296	488	1159
	SD	691	251	365	719
Fe	$\bar{X}$	14.4	4.5	15.6	14.8
	SD	9.8	2.8	7.8	4.0
Vitamins (mg)					
B_1	$\bar{X}$	1.57	0.51	1.53	1.64
	SD	0.89	0.45	0.83	0.58
B_2	$\bar{X}$	1.64	0.44	1.45	1.76
	SD	0.88	0.19	0.77	0.65
PP	$\bar{X}$	18.0	7.1	24.7	23.4
	SD	11.6	8.6	9.3	8.5
C	$\bar{X}$	17.4	23.5	88.8	26.8
	SD	19.3	12	36.7	20.9

at the end of the prenatal period, during breast feeding), weaning, and puberty, which can significantly modify the later development of a number of characteristics of an organism. Therefore, proper regimes of nutrition and exercise should be introduced already during these early periods of life. A search for and an introduction of scientifically based measures concerning diet and exercise in early life seems to be a very promising approach to the achievements of the optimal somatic development, body composition, nutritional status, and physical performance levels.

As regards the energy and food component recommendations, an individual approach based on the complex evaluation of the athlete at any age, level, and specialization seems to be indispensable. The evaluation should include an individual's history, since the impact of nutrition is both immediate and delayed. Only in such a way can a diet contribute positively to the achievement of the best physical performance both in recreational and championship sports.

References

Brozek, J., & Schürch, B. (1984). Malnutrition and behaviour: Critical assessment of key issues. Nestle Foundation, Lausanne, Switzerland.

Dobbing, J. (1984). Infant nutrition and later achievement. *Nutr. Rev.*, **42**, 1-7.

Energy and protein requirements. Report of a joint FAO/WHO/UNU Expert Consultation. World Health Organization, Geneva. Technical Report Services 724; 1985.

Faltová, E., Mráz, M., Pařizková, J., & Sedivý, J. (1985). Physical activity of different intensities and the development of myocardial resistance to injury. *Physiol. bohemoslov.*, **34**, 289-296.

Faltová, E., Parizková, J., Mráz, M., Sedivý, J., & Spátová, M. (1983). Influence of motor activity on the development of isoprenaline induced heart lesions. *Physiol. bohemoslov.*, **32**, 203-209.

Hejda, S., Vigner, J., Urbánek, J., Jirka, Z., Kocová, J., Sperlingová, L., & Voldánová, M. (1978). Recommended allowances of nutrition and individual foodstuffs for champion athletes. Association for Rational Nutrition, Prague.

Koch, J. (1976). *Total baby development*. Wyden Books, Ridgefield, CT.

Pařizková, J. (1978a). Body composition and lipid metabolism in relation to nutrition and exercise. In J. Pařizková & V.A. Rogozkin (Eds.), *Nutrition, physical fitness and health*. International Series on Sports Sciences, Vol. 7, University Park Press, Baltimore, 61-75.

Pařizková, J. (1978b). The impact of daily work load during pregnancy and/or postnatal life on the heart microstructure of rat male offspring. *Basic Res. Cardiol.*, **73**, 433-441.

Pařizková, J. (1979). Cardiac microstructure in female and male offspring of exercised rat mothers. *Acta Anat.*, **104**, 382-387.

Pařizková, J. (1983). Nutrition, body composition and fitness in old men. In J.C. Szomogyi & F. Fidanza (Eds.), *Nutritional problems of the elderly*. Bibl. Nutr. Dieta, 33, Karger, Basel, 31-41.

Pařizková, J. (1985a). Adaptation of functional capacity and exercise. In K. Blater & J.C. Waterlaw (Eds.), *Nutritional adaptation in man*. John Libbey, London and Paris, 127-139.

Pařizková, J. (1985b). *Body composition and nutrition of different types of athletes*. In T.G. Taylor & N.K. Jenkins (Eds.), Proceedings of the XIII International Congress of Nutrition, 1985, John Libbey, London and Paris, 309-311.

Pařizková, J. (1987). *Nutrition, energy expenditure and exercise*. In A. Tsopana & J. Poortmans (Eds.), Proceedings of the 3rd International Course on Physiological Biochemistry of Exercise and Training, Athens, Hellenic Sports Research Institute, Olympic Center of Athens, 1987, 239-255.

Pařizková, J., Bunc, V., Sprynarová, S., Macková, E., & Heller, J. (1987). Body composition, aerobic capacity, ventilatory threshold and food intake in different sports. *Ann. Sports Med.*, **3**, 171-177.

Pařizková, J., & Faltová, E. (1970). Physical activity, body fat and experimental cardiac necrosis. *Br. J. Nutr.*, **24**, 3-10.

Pařizková, J., Faltová, E., Mráz, M., & Spátová, M. (1982). Growth, food intake, motor activity and experimental cardiac necrosis in early malnourished male rats. *Ann. Nutr. Metab.*, **26**, 121-128.

Pařizková, J., Franková, S., Spátová, M., & Petrásek, R. (1980). Spontaneous motor activity, energy cost of growth and lipid metabolism in the liver in male rats with early protein energy malnutrition. *Baroda J. Nutr.*, **7**, 49-54.

Pařizková, J., Macková, E., Kábele, J., Macková, J., & Skopková, M. (1986). Body composition, food intake, cardiorespiratory fitness, blood lipids and physiological development in highly active and inactive preschool children. *Human Biol.*, **58**, 261-273.

Pařizková, J., & Petrásek, R. (1979). The impact of daily work load during pregnancy on lipid metabolism in the liver of the offspring. In J.C. Szomogyi & J.F. de Wijn (Eds.), *Nutritional aspects of physical performance*. Bibl. Nutr. Dieta, No. 27, Karger, Basel, 57-64.

Pařizková, J., Petrásek, R., & Franková, S. (1979). The impact of reduced energy and protein intake at the beginning of life on growth, spontaneous motor activity and lipid metabolism in male rats. *The Ind. J. Nutr. Dietet.*, **16**, 412-416.

Pařizková, J., Sonka, J., & Melicharová, E. (1985). Nahrungsaufnahme, Körperbau, Körperzusammensetzung und Lipidstoffwechsel bei erwachsenen Teilnehmern am Freizeitund Erholungssport. In J. Pařizková (Ed.), *Ernährung, körperliche Leistungsfähigkeit und Gesundheit*. Johann Ambrosius Barth, Leipzig, 130-139.

Widdowson, E.M. (1962). Nutritional individuality. *Proc. Nutr. Soc.*, **21**, 121-128.

Hypothalamic Control of Energy Metabolism

T. Shimazu

Department of Medical Biochemistry, School of Medicine, Ehime University, Shigenobu, Japan

Exercise is perhaps the most powerful stimulus for increasing the metabolic rate, and the energy required for physical work derives from the oxidation of carbohydrate or fat. At the onset of exercise, signals are transmitted from the brain not only to the muscles to cause muscle contractions but also to the autonomic centers to initiate mass sympathetic discharge into visceral organs. The activation of the sympathetic nervous system leads to glucose output from the liver and fat mobilization from the adipose tissue in conjunction with increased levels of plasma glucagon and catecholamines. It has been established that these metabolic alterations are controlled by the autonomic center of the hypothalamus. Evidence for this has come mainly from studies on changes in the metabolic parameters in response to direct electrical and chemical stimulations or electrolytic lesions of the specific locations within the hypothalamus (Shimazu, 1979, 1981, 1986, 1987). In this paper, I will review briefly our previous studies on the subject.

Reciprocal Function of the Hypothalamus in Metabolic Control

In the hypothalamus there are groups of nerve cells or nuclei that can be roughly divided structurally and functionally into the medial and the lateral hypothalamic areas at the boundary of the fornix. Although the medial hypothalamus actually contains several nuclei, the ventromedial hypothalamic nucleus (VMH) has a central function. The lateral hypothalamus is composed of the lateral hypothalamic nucleus (LH), the cells of which are diffusely scattered among the upward and downward nerve fibers.

Previous studies have revealed that the VMH and LH act reciprocally in several regulatory functions. For regulation of food intake, for instance, the VMH is believed to act as the satiety center, while the LH acts as the feeding center (Oomura, 1973). With respect to regulatory influences on autonomic nerves, the VMH is considered to belong to the sympathetic system and the LH to the parasympathetic system (Ban, 1975). In general, the functions of the VMH and LH in metabolic regulation also seem to be reciprocal, particularly in the regulation of carbohydrate metabolism (Shimazu, 1979, 1981, 1986, 1987). Thus, electrical and chemical stimulations of the VMH cause glycogenolysis and enhance gluconeogenesis in the liver to produce hyperglycemia, whereas stimulations of the LH promote glycogenesis and inhibit gluconeogenesis in the liver. Stimulations of the VMH elicit glucagon secretion from the pancreas, while stimulations of the LH induce selective release of insulin. This hypothalamic modulation of endocrine pancreas can affect glucose metabolism in the liver.

The reciprocal functions of the VMH and LH in metabolic regulation parallel those of the sympathetic and parasympathetic nerves (Shimazu, 1983). Thus, the signals emanating from some VMH neurons are presumed to travel caudally through the midbrain and pons, interact with neurons residing in the central gray substance of the brainstem, and continue through the medulla by polysynaptic pathways to the intermediolateral cell column of the thoracolumbar spinal cord and then to the splanchnic nerves that innervate various abdominal viscera. Information from some of the neurons in the LH may travel through the dorsal motor nucleus of the vagus and the nucleus ambiguus of the medulla and connect with the vagus nerves that distribute to a wide variety of thoracic and abdominal organs. Hence, we proposed that this functional organization of the VMH–splanchnic sympathetic nerve and LH–vagus parasympathetic nerve pathways can mediate efferent neuronal effects on peripheral metabolism (Shimazu, 1981, 1983).

Hypothalamic Control of Carbohydrate Metabolism

The VMH and LH act in a reciprocal manner on glycogen metabolism in the liver to provide nearly instantaneous effects on glucoregulation. The first evidence of this was obtained from studies of changes in liver glycogen metabolism after electrical stimulation of these hypothalamic nuclei (Shimazu et al., 1966, 1978). Stimulation of the VMH causes glucose output from the liver by rapid activation of glycogen phosphorylase, the enzyme catalyzing the rate-limiting step in glycogenolysis, and results in hyperglycemia and a marked reduction in the liver glycogen content. Stimulation of the LH, in contrast, leads to hepatic glycogenesis by activation of the key enzyme, glycogen synthetase, and tends to decrease the blood glucose level.

The question of whether these hypothalamic effects on hepatic glycogen metabolism originate from specific neurons in the VMH and LH or from nerve fibers traversing these loci has been resolved by using chemical stimulation, which has, in addition, provided some characteristics of chemical coding of the metabolic responses (Matsushita & Shimazu, 1980; Shimazu et al., 1976). Microinjection of norepinephrine into the VMH selectively induces rapid activation of glycogen phosphorylase in the liver and mimics the changes observed after electrical stimulation. The concentrations required, approximately 5×10^{-10} moles, are well within the physiological range. On the other hand, microinjection of acetylcholine into the LH specifically causes marked activation of glycogen synthetase in the liver, an effect that can be blocked by previous microinjection of anticholinergic agents such as atropine and scopolamine. Systemic injection of N-methylatropine also inhibits the hypothalamic effect of acetylcholine, demonstrating that both the central and peripheral mechanisms of the regulatory system are under cholinergic influences.

The hypothalamic control of carbohydrate metabolism involves neural–hormonal and direct neural mechanisms. Indeed, glycogen breakdown and synthesis in the liver are influenced by catecholamines, glucagon, and insulin. Secretion of these hormones has been shown to be modulated by the hypothalamus and the autonomic nerves (Shimazu, 1986, 1987): Sympathetic innervation of the pancreas, via the VMH-splanchnic nerve connection, stimulates the release of glucagon and inhibits insulin release. Conversely the parasympathetic innervation of the pancreas, via the LH-vagal connection, enhances the release of insulin. It has been proposed by us that the hypothalamus has a dual mechanism of control over liver glycogen metabolism and glucose homeostasis. One mechanism is the neural–hormonal regulation of glycogenolysis and glycogenesis, which involves neural stimulation of the release of pancreatic hormones and of adrenomedullary catecholamines, and is responsible for prolongation or consolidation of metabolic changes rather than for their initiation. The other mechanism is by direct innervation of the liver, via the "VMH-splanchnic" and the "LH-vagus nerve pathways," which directly control the enzymes metabolizing glycogen in the liver and thus are responsible for the initial and fine regulation of metabolic changes (Shimazu, 1981, 1983).

The first evidence that hepatic carbohydrate metabolism is under direct control of hepatic sympathetic innervation was obtained in 1965, when we demonstrated rapid and marked increases in the activities of hepatic glycogenolytic enzymes (phosphorylase and glucose 6-phosphatase), with a concomitant decrease in the liver glycogen content after electrical stimulation of the peripheral end of the left splanchnic nerve of rabbits (Shimazu & Fukuda, 1965). Since the effects of splanchnic nerve stimulation still persisted after removal of the adrenals or of the pancreas, which also receive sympathetic innervation, it was concluded that the release of either epinephrine from the adrenal or of glucagon from the pancreas was not necessary for the rapid increases in hepatic glycogenolytic enzymes in response to splanchnic nerve stimulation, and that these effects were directly dependent on hepatic sympathetic innervation (Shimazu, 1981, 1983).

Recently progress has been made in studies on neural regulation of hepatic glucose metabolism by stimulating the perivascular nerve bundles (hepatic nerves) of the liver perfused in situ (Beckh et al., 1987; Shimazu, 1983). This perfusion technique makes it possible to study a completely isolated organ whose efferent nerve supply to the liver has been kept intact and where any possible effects of the endocrine pancreas and other humoral factors can be excluded. In this hepatic nerve–liver preparation perfused in situ, electrical stimulation of the postganglionic sympathetic nerve bundles resulted in rapid increases of glucose and lactate outputs and an activation of hepatic phosphorylase. The possible complication that nerve stimulation induces decreased portal flow under constant pressure owing to an increase in vascular resistance and a microcirculatory alteration has been overcome by pharmacological means. The use of an irreversible α-antagonist, phenoxybenzamine, almost completely prevented the hemodynamic changes resulting from sympathetic nerve stimulation without affecting such metabolic alterations as the rapid activation of liver phosphorylase and enhancement of glucose output (Shimazu, 1983). It thus appears that hemodynamic and metabolic effects of nerve stimulation can be separated, and that the metabolic effects of nerve stimulation cannot be ascribed merely to changes in portal flow. Therefore, these findings can be taken to indicate that glycogenolysis and glucose output in the liver are directly regulated by the intrinsic sympathetic innervation of hepatocytes.

Evidence was also obtained for a role of parasympathetic nerves in regulating glycogen synthesis in the liver (Shimazu, 1971; Shimazu & Fujimoto, 1971). The activity of liver glycogen synthetase, the rate-limiting enzyme involved in converting glucose 6-phosphate to glycogen, was greatly increased by electrical stimulation of the peripheral end of the vagus nerve, but was slightly decreased by splanchnic nerve stimulation. The increase in enzyme activity on vagal stimulation was shown to be due to conversion of the physiologically inactive form of the enzyme to the active form. This effect of vagal stimulation was not eliminated by previous pancreatectomy, indicating that the effect was not secondary to insulin released from the pancreas, but was due mainly to direct neural control. However, the effect was completely counteracted by simultaneous stimulation of the splanchnic nerve. The activation of glycogen synthetase induced by vagal stimulation actually reflects an increased rate of glycogen synthesis in the liver. On vagal stimulation, the rate of incorporation of radioactive glucose into liver glycogen in vivo was markedly (about fivefold) increased whereas, on splanchnic nerve stimulation, the opposite effect was observed (Shimazu & Fujimoto, 1971).

Hypothalamic Control of Lipid Metabolism

There is some evidence that the central nervous system, especially the hypothalamus, is involved in regulation of lipolysis or fat mobilization from adipose tissues (Shimazu, 1981, 1986). Our previous studies (Takahashi & Shimazu, 1981) showed that electrical stimulation of the VMH caused lipolysis in anesthetized rats, detected by marked increases in the plasma levels of glycerol and free fatty acids (FFA), whereas electrical stimulation of the LH had no appreciable effect on the concentrations of plasma glycerol and FFA. To determine the relative importance of the sympathetic nervous system and the adrenal medulla for VMH-induced lipolysis in rats, the effects of adrenodemedullation and adrenergic blockade were studied (Takahashi & Shimazu, 1981). Bilateral adrenodemedullation did not prevent the lipolytic response to VMH stimulation, although it reduced slightly (about 20-30%) the increment of plasma glycerol and FFA. However, the lipolytic response was completely blocked by previous treatment of the animals with hexamethonium (ganglion blocker) or propranolol (β-adrenergic blocker), but not with phentolamine (α-blocker). These results suggest that the sympathetic innervation of adipose tissue through a β-adrenoceptor mechanism is the dominant factor involved in VMH-induced lipolysis.

Neuronal control of lipid synthesis has been rather neglected until recently. We have investigated the effect of hypothalamic stimulation on the rate of lipid synthesis in brown (BAT) and white adipose tissue (WAT) and the liver of rats by measuring the incorporation of tritium from ^3H_2O into fatty acids in vivo (Shimazu & Takahashi, 1980). The rate of fatty acid synthesis in control rats was much greater in the interscapular BAT than in the parametrial and retroperitoneal WAT. With electrical stimulation of the VMH, the rate increased (about 2.5 times that of unstimulated controls) in BAT, but not in WAT or the liver. Electrical stimulation of the LH, however, did not appreciably affect fatty acid synthesis in any of the three tissues. Electrical stimulation of the VMH was also shown to increase markedly the rate of conversion of ^{14}C-glucose into lipid fractions (including total lipids, fatty acids, glyceride glycerol and phospholipids) in interscapular BAT, but not in parametrial or retroperitoneal WAT. Conversely, on VMH stimulation, the synthesis of these lipid fractions from glucose in the liver decreased slightly. Again, electrical stimulation of the LH had no such effect.

These results indicate that stimulation of the VMH enhances lipogenesis in BAT preferentially. This effect is probably mediated by sympathetic innervation of BAT, because the VMH is presumed to be a hypothalamic component of the sympathetic nervous system. Brown adipose tissue has abundant sympathetic innervation which form nest-like networks around every fat cell, whereas WAT has no sympathetic fibers in direct contact with fat cells except those related to the blood vessels. This difference in sympathetic innervation of BAT and WAT possibly reflects the differential effects of VMH stimulation on lipogenesis observed in these two adipose tissues. Indeed, when the sympathetic nerves entering the interscapular BAT were sectioned, the increased rates of fatty acid and glyceride glycerol syntheses after VMH stimulation were suppressed almost completely (Minokoshi et al., 1986). These findings, coupled with the previous observation of increased lipolysis in adipose tissue after stimulation of the VMH, suggest that both the breakdown and resynthesis, that is the turnover, of triglycerides in BAT, but not in WAT, are accelerated by stimulation of the VMH and the sympathetic nerves. The increased turnover of triglycerides leads to enhanced fatty acid oxidation in mitochondria and resultant heat production unique to brown fat cells, which comprises a significant component of energy expenditure (Shimazu, 1986).

Conclusion

During exercise, activity in motor centers may evoke an arousal of the VMH neurons, which then increase the sympathetic outflow to the liver, WAT, BAT, adrenal medulla and pancreas. In the liver, glycogen breakdown is initiated and the resultant glucose is rapidly utilized by the muscles and other tissues, while lipid synthesis is suppressed. Increased secretion of pancreatic glucagon also contributes to glucose output from the liver. In WAT, the increased sympathetic outflow induces fat mobilization in cooperation with catecholamines released from the adrenal medulla, which contributes to ATP production and energy supply to other tissues through mitochondrial oxidation of fatty acids. In BAT, increased sympathetic activity accelerates triglyceride turnover by stimulating the fatty acid synthesis and breakdown cycle, which leads to enhanced fatty acid oxidation and heat production in mitochondria unique to this tissue. It thus appears that the VMH is importantly involved in both energy supply and energy expenditure of the body by regulating carbohydrate and lipid metabolism in the liver and adipose tissues.

References

Ban, T. (1975). Fiber connections in the hypothalamus and some autonomic functions. *Pharmacol. Biochem. Behav.*, **3**(Suppl. 1), 3-13.

Beckh, K., Beuers, U., Engelhardt, R., & Jungermann, K. (1987). Mechanism of action of sympathetic hepatic nerves on carbohydrate metabolism in perfused rat liver. *Biol. Chem. Hoppe-Seyler*, **368**, 379-386.

Matsushita, H., & Shimazu, T. (1980). Chemical coding of the hypothalamic neurones in metabolic control II. Norepinephrine-sensitive neurones and glycogen breakdown in liver. *Brain Res.*, **183**, 79-87.

Minokoshi, Y., Saito, M., & Shimazu, T. (1986). Sympathetic denervation impairs responses of brown adipose tissue to VMH stimulation. *Am. J. Physiol.*, **251**, R1005-R1008.

Oomura, Y. (1973). Central mechanism of feeding. In M. Kotani (Ed.), *Advances in biophysics*, Vol. 5. University of Tokyo Press, Tokyo, 65-142.

Shimazu, T. (1971). Regulation of glycogen metabolism in liver by the autonomic nervous system. V. Activation of glycogen synthetase by vagal stimulation. *Biochim. Biophys. Acta*, **252**, 28-38.

Shimazu, T. (1979). Nervous control of peripheral metabolism. *Acta Physiol. Pol.*, **30**(Suppl. 18), 1-18.

Shimazu, T. (1981). Central nervous system regulation of liver and adipose tissue metabolism. *Diabetologia*, **20**, 343-356.

Shimazu, T. (1983). Reciprocal innervation of the liver: Its significance in metabolic control. In A.J. Szabo (Ed.), *Advances in metabolic disorders, Vol. 10, CNS regulation of carbohydrate metabolism*. Academic Press, New York, 355-384.

Shimazu, T. (1986). Neuronal control of intermediate metabolism. In S.L. Lightman & B.J. Everitt (Eds.), *Neuroendocrinology*. Blackwell, Oxford, 304-340.

Shimazu, T. (1987). Neuronal regulation of hepatic glucose metabolism in mammals. *Diabetes/Metabolism Rev.*, **3**, 185-206.

Shimazu, T., & Fujimoto, T. (1971). Regulation of glycogen metabolism in liver by the autonomic nervous system. IV. Neural control of glycogen biosynthesis. *Biochim. Biophys. Acta*, **252**, 18-27.

Shimazu, T., & Fukuda, A. (1965). Increased activities of glycogenolytic enzymes in liver after splanchnic-nerve stimulation. *Science*, **150**, 1607-1608.

Shimazu, T., & Takahashi, A. (1980). Stimulation of hypothalamic nuclei has differential effects on lipid synthesis in brown and white adipose tissue. *Nature*, **284**, 62-63.

Shimazu, T., Fukuda, A., & Ban, T. (1966). Reciprocal influence of the ventromedial and lateral hypothalamic nuclei on blood glucose level and liver glycogen content. *Nature*, **210**, 1178-1179.

Shimazu, T., Matsushita, H., & Ishikawa, K. (1976). Cholinergic stimulation of the rat hypothalamus: Effects on liver glycogen synthesis. *Science*, **194**, 535-536.

Shimazu, T., Matsushita, H., & Ishikawa, K. (1978). Hypothalamic control of liver glycogen metabolism in adult and aged rats. *Brain Res.*, **144**, 343-352.

Takahashi, A., & Shimazu, T. (1981). Hypothalamic regulation of lipid metabolism in the rat: Effect of hypothalamic stimulation on lipolysis. *J. Auton. Nerv. Syst.*, **4**, 195-205.

Factors Affecting Skeletal Muscle Sensitivity to Insulin

L. Budohoski, R.A.J. Challiss, and E.A. Newsholme

Department of Applied Physiology, Medical Research Centre, Polish Academy of Sciences, Warsaw, Poland; Department of Pharmacology, Medical Sciences Building, University of Leicester, Leicester, U.K.; and Department of Biochemistry, University of Oxford, Oxford, U.K.

Insulin resistance is a state in which higher than normal concentration of the hormone is required to produce a given biological effect (Kahan, 1978). This could be caused by presence of antibodies to the hormone, production of abnormal and less effective insulin or decreased response of the target tissues to insulin (Olefsky et al., 1982). In the vast majority of cases of obesity and non-insulin-dependent diabetes mellitus, the latter problem is most relevant. It is known that in both these cases there is a decreased number of insulin receptors present in target tissues (Olefsky, 1976); however, present evidence would suggest that the post-receptor defects are primarily responsible for the resistance of target tissues to insulin (for reviews see Kahan, 1978; Olefsky et al., 1982). The precise nature or locus of these defects is at present unknown. Nevertheless, such lesions are considered to be primarily responsible for reduced ability of an affected individual to regulate blood glucose concentration.

Adenosine, a metabolite which has been known for many years to profoundly influence metabolism, particularly tissue perfusion (Berne, 1963, 1980; Fredholm & Sollevi, 1986), has been shown to potentiate the effects of insulin and attenuate the effects of catecholamines on glucose transport and lipolysis in white adipose tissue (Gliemann et al., 1985; Green & Newsholme, 1979; Shwabe et al., 1974; Trost & Stock, 1977). The physiological role of adenosine as a modulator of insulin action in skeletal muscle has not received enough attention.

A method for studying sensitivity of glucose utilization by skeletal muscles in vitro has been previously described (Challiss et al., 1983; Crettaz et al., 1980). In brief, this entails dissection of soleus muscle from Wistar rats (160-180 g) and longitudinal preparation of muscles to produce 30 to 35 mg muscle strips which are attached to metal springs to maintain the muscles under a tension approximating that observed in vivo. Soleus muscle strips are incubated for an initial 30-min period, to allow recovery from the preparation procedure, in Krebs-Ringer bicarbonate buffer containing 1.5% deffated albumin, 5.5 mM glucose, pyruvate, succinate, and glutamate (see Challiss et al., 1983). Muscle strips are then transferred to fresh medium containing glucose as the sole metabolized substrate and various concentrations of insulin (1-10000 μU/ml). Rate of lactate formation can be measured spectrophotometrically; however, to allow rates of glycogen synthesis and CO_2 production to be determined [U-^{14}C]glucose is added to the incubation medium; similarly, radiolabelled 3-o-methylglucose or 2-deoxyglucose may be added at tracer concentrations to follow the rates of glucose transport and/or phosphorylation (Challiss et al., 1986). In skeletal muscle, insulin stimulates the rate of glycogen synthesis and glucose transport (Randle & Morgan, 1962), and the same is true for the stripped soleus muscle preparation incubated in vitro (Espinal et al., 1983). The mean insulin sensitivity of both these processes to insulin (i.e., the hormone concentration producing half-maximal effect) is 100 μU/ml (Budohoski et al., 1984a; Challiss et al., 1983; Espinal et al., 1983).

In such muscle preparation, the reduction of endogenously produced adenosine to a very low concentration by addition of the enzyme adenosine deaminase (ADA, which is known to immediately convert adenosine to inosine), has a marked effect on the insulin sensitivity of glucose transport. Thus, addition of ADA reduces the concentration of insulin required to produce a half-maximal effect on glucose transport to approximately 10 μU/ml (Challiss et al., 1987; Espinal et al., 1983). Moreover, it has been shown that this apparent hormone-modulatory action of adenosine is occurring via adenosine receptors (Budohoski et al., 1984a). An addition of the adenosine receptor agonist 2-chloroadenosine to the incubation medium in a final concentration of 20 μM markedly decreases the sensitivity of glucose utilization, whereas an addition of the adenosine receptor antagonist 8-phenyltheophylline (2 μM) markedly increases sensitivity of glucose utilization by the soleus muscle to insulin (Budohoski et al., 1984a). It should be noted, however, that changing of the adenosine concentration or addition of either adenosine receptor antagonist or agonist does not influence the sensitivity of the glycogen synthesis to insulin.

Results obtained using the soleus muscle (which is composed of > 85% type I muscle fibers) have been confirmed using the extensor digitorum longus (which is composed of 50% type IIa and 50% IIb muscle fibers) and epitrochlearis muscle (composed predominantly of white fiber type), while in diaphragm, adenosine does not appear to have any insulin-modulatory action (Challiss et al., 1987; Leighton et al., in press). Under the conditions of identical investigations, adenosine was found to be present intra- and extra-cellularly (Lozeman et al., 1987) and the concentration of adenosine appears to exert a modulatory influence on the insulin-stimulated rate of glucose transport. The next question was whether physiological or pathological changes in the insulin sensitivity of the skeletal muscles can be influenced by changes in the effectiveness of adenosine. It was found that cold exposure at 4 °C for 2 to 7 days causes an increase of the sensitivity of glucose transport to insulin in skeletal muscles. This physiological adaptation can be reversed by addition in vitro of chloroadenosine (Budohoski et al., 1984b). In contrast, sucrose feeding (Budohoski et al., 1984c) causes a decrease in the sensitivity of glucose transport into skeletal muscle to insulin and this can be reversed by addition in vitro of ADA or adenosine-receptor antagonists (Budohoski et al., 1984c).

The genetically obese Zucker rat is hyperinsulinaemic and its adipose tissue, liver, and muscles display a dramatic decrease in insulin sensitivity of a number of metabolic processes (Crettaz et al., 1980); therefore, the obese Zucker rat has been extensively used as a model of noninsulin dependent diabetes. In skeletal muscles of Zucker rats both glucose transport and glycogen synthesis show a marked insulin resistance (Challiss et al., 1984; Crettaz et al., 1980), but only the sensitivity of glucose transport to insulin can be improved by in vitro addition of adenosine-receptor antagonist 8-phenyltheophylline (Challiss et al., 1984). The findings described above make a strong case for the hypothesis that alterations in the steady-state concentration of adenosine at the skeletal muscle adenosine receptor, and/or an adaptive change in the adenosine receptor, may play a role in the pathophysiological modulation of peripheral insulin sensitivity in vitro. However, the proof of this hypothesis will require measurements of adenosine concentration within the microenvironment of adenosine receptor and full characterization of the kinetic properties of adenosine receptors present in skeletal muscles. A common feature of conditions under which insulin sensitivity is improved (e.g., cold exposure, exercise) is an increase in the circulating catecholamines, whereas the decreased insulin sensitivity tends to be associated with normal or reduced levels of blood catecholamines.

Acute administration of adrenaline in vivo decreases the sensitivity of glucose uptake by peripheral tissues to insulin (Deibert & DeFronzo, 1980; Sacca et al., 1982). Similar effect has been shown in isolated soleus muscle in vitro and has been demonstrated to be due to adrenaline-stimulated glycogenolysis, increasing the concentrations of hexose monophosphates in the cell with the consequent inhibition of hexokinase activity and possibly glucose transport (Challiss et al., 1986; Chiasson et al., 1981). It has recently been shown that sustained elevation of blood adrenaline concentration for about 5 days has a biphasic effect on skeletal muscle insulin sensitivity. Following the initial decrease of the sensitivity to insulin there is a significant increase in insulin sensitivity compared to control animals after 120 hours of hyperadrenalinemia (Budohoski et al., 1987). Similarly, chronic administration of the beta-adrenoreceptor agonist tetrabutaline improves insulin sensitivity (Scheidegger et al., 1984a) in experimental animals, and chronic treatment of genetically obese Zucker rats with a novel beta-adrenoreceptor agonist (BRL 26830A) reverses the insulin resistance observed in these animals (Smith et al., 1985), and the improvement in insulin sensitivity can be demonstrated in skeletal muscle (Challiss et al., 1985).

Clearly, further work is required to establish whether adenosine modulation of insulin action may depend on the plasma concentration of catecholamines since a number of other possibilities exist to explain the effect of catecholamines on peripheral insulin sensitivity (e.g., desensitization of muscle adrenoreceptors; Scheidegger et al., 1984b), or catecholamine-induced changes in thyroid hormones (Muller & Seitz, 1984; Scheidegger et al., 1984a). However, it should be noted that chronic adrenalinaemia leads to a specific adaptive response in the sensitivity of glucose transport process to insulin, with no apparent affect on glycogen synthase (Budohoski et al., 1987), a feature common to the action of adenosine in skeletal muscle. This has led to our current working hypothesis that the chronic elevation of catecholamine concentration may modify the steady-state interstitial concentration of adenosine in skeletal muscle or alter the properties of muscle adenosine receptors, thereby changing the sensitivity of glucose transport process to insulin. Irrespective of the physiological importance of adenosine as a hormone modulator, the studies summarized here provide evidence that adenosine-receptor agonists and antagonists can alter skeletal muscle insulin sensitivity. Therefore, it is conceivable that rational drug design of specific adenosine-receptor antagonist may provide a novel approach to the treatment of peripheral insulin resistance in a number of disease states.

Acknowledgments

The authors gratefully acknowledge the financial support of the Wellcome Trust and the British Diabetic Association. This work was also partly supported by the Polish Central Programme for Basic Research 06-02. III.

References

Berne, R.M. (1963). Cardiac nucleotides in hypoxia: A possible role in regulation of coronary blood flow. Am. J. Physiol., 204, 317-322.

Berne, R.M. (1980). The role of adenosine in the regulation of coronary blood flow. Circ. Res., 47, 807-813.

Budohoski, L., Challiss, R.A.J., McManus, B., & Newsholme, E.A. (1984a). Effects of analogues of adenosine and methylxantines on insulin sensitivity in soleus muscle of the rat. FEBS Lett., 167, 1-4.

Budohoski, L., Challiss, R.A.J., Lozeman, F.J., McManus, B., & Newsholme, E.A. (1984b). Increased insulin sensitivity in soleus muscle from cold-exposed rats: Reversal by an adenosine-receptor agonist. FEBS Lett., 175, 402-406.

Budohoski, L., Challiss, R.A.J., Cooney, G.J., McManus, B., & Newsholme, E.A. (1984c). Reversal of dietary-induced insulin resistance in muscle of the rat by adenosine deaminase and an adenosine-receptor antagonist. Biochem. J., 224, 327-330.

Budohoski, L., Challiss, R.A.J., Dubaniewicz, A., Kaciuba-Uścïłko, H., Leighton, B., Lozeman, F.J., Nazar, K., Newsholme, E.A., & Porta, S. (1987). Effects of prolonged elevation of plasma adrenaline concentration *in vivo* on insulin sensitivity in soleus muscle of the rat. *Biochem. J., 244,* 655-660.

Challiss, R.A.J., Espinal, J., & Newsholme, E.A. (1983). Insulin sensitivity of rates of glycolysis and glycogen synthesis in stripped soleus, epitrochlearis, and hemi-diaphragm muscles isolated from sedentary rats. *Biosci. Rep.* 3, 675-679.

Challiss, R.A.J., Budohoski, L., McManus, B., & Newsholme, E.A. (1984). Effects of an adenosine-receptor antagonist on insulin-resistance in soleus muscle from obese Zucker rats. *Biochem. J., 221,* 915-917.

Challiss, R.A.J., Budohoski, L., Newsholme, E.A., Sennit, M.V., & Cawthorne, M.A. (1985). Effect of a novel thermogenic β-adrenoreceptor agonist (BRL 2630) on insulin resistance in soleus muscle from obese Zucker rats. *Biochem. Biophys. Res. Commun., 128,* 928-935.

Challiss, R.A.J., Lozeman, F.J., Leighton, B., & Newsholme, E.A. (1986). Effects of the β-adrenoreceptor agonist isoprenaline on insulin sensitivity in soleus muscle of the rat. *Biochem. J., 233,* 377-381.

Challiss, R.A.J., Leighton, B., Lozeman, F.J., & Newsholme, E.A. (1987). The hormone-modulatory effects of adenosine in skeletal muscle. In Gerlach & Becker (Eds.), *Topics and perspectives in adenosine research 1987.* Springer-Verlag, Berlin, Heidelberg, 275-285.

Chiasson, J-L., Shikama, H., Chu, D.T.W., & Exton, J.H. (1981). Inhibitory effects of epinephrine on insulin-stimulated glucose uptake by rat skeletal muscle. *J. Clin. Invest., 68,* 706-713.

Crettaz, M., Prentki, M., Zaninetti, D., & Jeanrenaud, B. (1980). Insulin resistance in soleus muscle from obese Zucker rats. *Biochem. J., 186,* 525-534.

Deibert, D.C., & DeFronzo, R.A. (1980). Epinephrine-induced insulin resistance in man. *J. Clin. Invest., 65,* 717-721.

Espinal, J., Challiss, R.A.J., & Newsholme, E.A. (1983). Effect of adenosine deaminase and adenosine analogue on insulin sensitivity in soleus muscle of the rat. *FEBS Lett., 158,* 103-106.

Fredholm, B.B., & Sollevi, A. (1986). Cardiovascular effects of adenosine. *Clin. Physiol., 6,* 1-21.

Gliemann, J., Bowes, S.B., Larsen, T.R., & Rees, W.D. (1985). The effect of catechola-mines and adenosine deaminase on the glucose transport system in rat adipocytes. *Biochim. Biophys. Acta., 845,* 373-379.

Green, A., & Newsholme, A.E. (1979). Sensitivity of glucose transport and lipolysis of adipocytes to insulin and the effects of some metabolites. *Biochem. J., 180,* 356-365.

Kahan, C.R. (1978). Insulin resistance, insulin sensitivity and insulin unresponsiveness: A necessary distinction. *Metabolism, 27*(Suppl. 2), 1893-1902.

Leighton, B., Lozeman, F.J., Vlachonikolis, I.G., Challiss, R.A.J., Pitcher, J.A., & Newsholme, E.A. (in press). Effects of adenosine deaminase on the sensitivity of glucose transport, glycolysis and glycogen synthesis to insulin in muscles of the rat. *Int. J. Biochem.*

Lozeman, F.J., Challiss, R.A.J., Leighton, B., & Newsholme, E.A. (1987). Effects of dipyridamol on adenosine concentration, insulin sensitivity and glucose utilization in soleus muscle of the rat. *Pflügers Arch., 410,* 192-197.

Muller, M.J., & Seitz, H.J. (1984). Thyroid hormone action on intermediatory metabolism. *Klin. Wochenschr., 62,* 11-18.

Olefsky, J.M., Kolterman, O.G., & Scarlett, J.A. (1982). Insulin action and resistance in obesity and noninsulin-dependent type II diabetes mellitus. *Am. J. Physiol., 243,* E15-E30.

Olefsky, J.M. (1976). The insulin receptor: Its role in insulin resistance in obesity and diabetes. *Diabetes, 25,* 1154-1165.

Randle, P.J., & Morgan, H.E. (1962). Regulation of glucose uptake by muscle. *Vitam. Horm., 20,* 199-250.

Sacca, L., Vigorito, C., Cicala, M., Ungaro, B., & Sherwin, R.S. (1982). Mechanisms of epinephrine-induced glucose intolerance in normal humans. *J. Clin. Invest., 69,* 284-293.

Scheidegger, K., Robbins, D.C., & Danforth, E. (1984a). Effects of chronic β-receptor stimulation on glucose metabolism. *Diabetes, 33,* 1144-1149.

Scheidegger, K., O'Connell, M., Robbins, D.C., & Danforth, E. (1984b). Effects of chronic β-receptor activity, energy expenditure and thyroid hormones. *J. Clin. Endocrinol. Metab., 58,* 895-903.

Schwabe, U., Schonhofer, P.S., & Ebert, R. (1974). Facilitation by adenosine of the action of insulin on the accumulation of cyclic AMP, lipolysis and glucose oxidation in isolated fat cells. *Eur. J. Biochem., 46,* 537-545.

Smith, S.A., Levy, A.L., Sennitt, M.V., Simson, D.L., & Cawthorne, M.A. (1985). Effects of BRL 26830, a novel β-adrenoreceptor agonist, on glucose tolerance, insulin sensitivity and glucose turnover in Zucker (fa/fa) rats. *Biochem. Pharmacol., 34,* 2425-2429.

Trost, T., & Stock, K. (1977). Effects of adenosine derivatives on cyclic AMP accumulation and lipolysis in rat adipocytes and on adenylate cyclase in adipocyte plasma membranes. *Naunyn Schmiedebergs Arch. Pharmacol., 229,* 33-40.

RESEARCH NOTES

Effects of Nonselective β-Adrenergic Receptor Blockade on Adenine Nucleotide Catabolism in Thigh Muscle During Maximal Exercise

B. Norman, E. Jansson, P. Kaiser, P.A. Tesch, A. Sollevi, and L. Kaijser

Department of Clinical Physiology, Karolinska Hospital and Department of Environmental Medicine and Pharmacology, Karolinska Institute, Stockholm, Sweden

The aim of the present study was to investigate the effects of β-adrenergic receptor blockade on muscle metabolism at the time of exhaustion at an incremental cycle ergometer test by analyzing the contents of adenine nucleotides and their degradation products in the thigh muscle. Six healthy trained men (mean $\pm$ SD of age, height, and weight: 22 $\pm$ 4 years, 184 $\pm$ 7 cm, and 78 $\pm$ 8 kg) were studied on two occasions and randomized in a double blind cross-over fashion. Subjects were given placebo (PL) or 80 mg propranolol (PR) (Inderal®). The drug was taken orally 105 min before exercise. Maximal exercise was performed on an electrically braked cycle ergometer that started at a power output corresponding to 70% of predicted individual maximal oxygen uptake ($\dot{V}O_2$max), and the load was increased by 30 W/min until exhaustion. Expired air was collected in Douglas bags at higher exercise intensities for determination of $\dot{V}O_2$max (Kaiser et al., 1986). Heart rate (HR) was calculated from ECG recordings. A muscle sample was obtained by a needle biopsy technique from the m. vastus lateralis within 15 s after cessation of the maximal exercise and analyzed for ATP, ADP, AMP, IMP, hypoxanthine (HPX), and uric acid (UA) (Norman et al., 1987). The study was approved by the Ethics Committee of the Karolinska Hospital.

$\dot{V}O_2$max and HR immediately prior to exhaustion with PL and PR were 4.5 $\pm$ 0.4 and 3.9 $\pm$ 0.4 L min^{-1} ($p < .01$) and 187 $\pm$ 5 and 138 $\pm$ 13 bpm ($p < .001$), respectively. Performance time decreased with PR from 419 $\pm$ 40 to 318 $\pm$ 29 s ($p < .01$). There were no significant differences between PL and PR at exhaustion in muscle ATP, ADP, AMP, IMP, and UA contents which were 21.3 $\pm$ 2.4, 4.14 $\pm$ 0.92, 0.32 $\pm$ 0.19, 2.70 $\pm$ 1.88 and 0.38 $\pm$ 0.17 respectively with PL and 21.2 $\pm$ 3.07, 3.89 $\pm$ 0.90, 0.36 $\pm$ 0.24, 3.31 $\pm$ 2.12 and 0.45 $\pm$ 0.18 mmol • Kg^{-1} dm with PR. HPX content was significantly higher with PR than PL (0.14 $\pm$ 0.09 vs 0.07 $\pm$ 0.07 mmol • kg $- 1_{dm}$, $p < 0.05$). The total adenine nucleotide content TAN (ATP + ADP + AMP) was not different between PL and PR (26.9 $\pm$ 2.3 vs 25.3 $\pm$ 4.3 mmol • kg$^{-1}_{dm}$). Energy charge ([ATP + 0.5 ADP]/TAN) was 0.91 $\pm$ 0.01 for both PL and PR. Only a few studies are reported regarding degradation products from the adenine nucleotides in human skeletal muscle (e.g., Sabina et al., 1984; Sahlin et al., 1978). The IMP levels at exhaustion found

125

in the present study are similar to those presented by Sahlin et al. (1978) after maximal exercise to exhaustion in healthy males.

HPX levels on patients performing short-term cycle exercise to exhaustion (Sabina et al., 1984) were comparable to those found after PL in the present study. Despite decreased performance time higher HPX content was shown with PR than with PL in the present study. This difference may be explained most likely by a lower leg blood flow (leading to decreased oxygen delivery and HPX wash-out) with β-blockade due to a lower cardiac output. It is very unlikely that the large decrease in maximal heart rate (from 187 to 138) could have been compensated for by a corresponding increase in stroke volume. Another possible reason for the higher HPX with PR could be a substrate deficiency. The glycogenolysis is thought to be retarded by β-blockade, as indicated by lowered G-6-P level (Kaiser et al., 1986) as is the lipolysis, which lowers the plasma free fatty acid concentration (Deacon, 1978). Consequently, there is probably a smaller amount of available substrate with β-blockade. This may impair the ATP regeneration capacity, thus increasing degradation products as HPX. An impaired ATP regeneration was also indicated by Kaiser et al. (1986) who demonstrated decreased muscle ATP and CP after exhaustive exercise with β-blockade. Brooke et al. (1983) showed in patients with phosphorylase deficiency (McArdle disease) an increased release of HPX from muscle to blood during exercise indicating a larger HPX production. These patients possess a substrate deficiency due to the inability to utilize muscle glycogen. Thus, to some extent, the substrate supply to the muscle appears to be similar after acute β-blockade and in patients suffering from McArdle disease.

Acknowledgments

This study was supported by grants from the Swedish Medical Research Council (No. 4494 and 7485) and the ICI-Pharma, Sweden.

References

Brooke, M.H., Patterson, V.H., & Kaiser, K.K. (1983). Hypoxanthine and McArdle disease: A clue to metabolic stress in working forearm. *Muscle & Nerve, 6*, 204-206.

Deacon, S.P. (1978). The effects of atenolol and propranolol upon lipolysis. *Br. J. Clin. Pharmacol., 5*, 123-125.

Kaiser, P., Tesch, P.A., Frisk-Holmberg, M., Juhlin-Dannfelt, A., & Kaijser, L. (1986). Effects of β_1-selective and non-selective β-blockade on work capacity and muscle metabolism. *Clin. Physiol., 6*, 197-207.

Norman, B., Sollevi, A., Kaijser, L., & Jansson, E. (1987). ATP breakdown products in human skeletal muscle during prolonged exercise to exhaustion. *Clin. Physiol, 7*, 503-509.

Sabina, R.L., Swain, J.L., Olanov, C.W., Bradley, W.G., Fishbein, W.N., Dimauro, S., & Holmes, E.W. (1984). Myoadenylate deaminase deficiency: Functional and metabolic abnormalities associated with disruption of the purine nucleotide cycle. *J. Clin. Invest., 73*, 720-730.

Sahlin, K., Palmskog, G., & Hultman, E. (1978). Adenine nucleotide and IMP contents of the quadriceps muscle in man after exercise. *Pflügers Arch., 374*, 193-198.

Fetal Metabolic Response to Mother's Exercise

M. Nowacka and J. Górski

Department of Clinical Physiology and Physiology, Medical School,
Białystok, Poland

There are some data indicating that exercise during pregnancy may affect fetal homeostasis. It is manifested by changes in pH, pO_2, pCO_2, concentration of glucose, and catecholamines in the fetal blood, as well as by alterations in fetal heart and respiratory rates. Some but not all authors found impaired development of the fetuses by training (Bonds & Delivoria-Papadopoulos, 1985; Górski, 1985; Mottola et al., 1983). The aim of the present study was to examine the effect of acute and chronic exercise during pregnancy on concentration of some metabolic compounds in the amniotic fluid and fetal liver.

Material and Methods

The experiments were carried out on female Wistar rats of body weight 200 g at the beginning of the study. They were kept with males and daily vaginal smears were taken. The first appearance of the sperm in the smear was considered as the first day of pregnancy. The pregnant rats were divided into two groups: I, untrained and II, trained. The rats of the second group were forced to run 2 h daily with the speed of 1000 m/h on a treadmill set at 10° incline. The untrained rats were familiarized with the treadmill by forcing them to run as above, 10 min daily, for six days preceding the final experiment. The rats of both groups were sacrificed on the 20th day of pregnancy.

Each group was divided into three subgroups: resting, exercising for 30 min, and exercising till exhaustion before being sacrificed. The rats were anesthetized with urethane administered intraperitoneally. The amniotic fluid was aspirated from several amnions and pulled. Then, the liver samples were taken from each fetus. The concentrations of compounds in the amniotic fluid were determined using conventional chemical or enzymatic (for urea) methods. The contents of glycogen and triglycerides in the fetal liver were determined as previously described (Górski, 1983). The mean differences between groups were evaluated using Student t test for unpaired data. The results are presented as means and standard deviations ($n = 10$).

Results

The number of fetuses in the sedentary (S) group was 11.3 ± 2.6, and in the trained (T) group was 10.8 ± 1.4; the average fetal body weight in S group was 2.3 ± 0.8 g and in T group 2.4 ± 0.8 g ($p > .05$). Time of running till exhaustion in S group was 128.4 ± 27.2 min, and in T group 170.0 ± 29.4 min ($p < .001$).

The concentrations of compounds determined are presented in Table 1. Thirty-min exercise had no significant effect on the concentration of either compound. Exercise till exhaustion reduced concentration of glucose and elevated concentration of urea in the amniotic

Table 1   Effect of Mother's Exercise on the Level of Different Compounds in the Amniotic Fluid and on Glycogen and Triglycerides in the Fetal Liver

Compound	Group	Rest	30 min	Exhaustion
			Exercise	
Amniotic fluid				
Glucose	S	2.64 ± 0.98	3.28 ± 0.93[a]	3.07 ± 0.61
(mmol · L⁻¹)	T	2.91 ± 1.10	2.40 ± 0.14	1.91 ± 0.74[a]
Protein	S	0.94 ± 0.32	0.73 ± 0.20	0.73 ± 0.21
(g · dl⁻¹)	T	0.78 ± 0.30	0.82 ± 0.13	0.77 ± 0.16
Cholesterol (total)	S	0.28 ± 0.10	0.37 ± 0.17	0.33 ± 0.08
(mmol · L⁻¹)	T	0.55 ± 0.18[d]	0.55 ± 0.06[c]	0.62 ± 0.09[d]
Creatinine	S	151.2 ± 42.3	112.3 ± 39.8	163.5 ± 31.8
(μmol · L⁻¹)	T	122.9 ± 15.0	109.6 ± 20.3	149.8 ± 59.2
Urea	S	7.17 ± 1.65	7.12 ± 2.07	8.74 ± 2.67
(mmol · L⁻¹)	T	5.41 ± 0.76	6.48 ± 1.63[c]	6.50 ± 1.22[a]
Uric acid	S	72.6 ± 36.9	110.7 ± 73.2	173.1 ± 71.4[b]
(μmol · L⁻¹)	T	99.4 ± 46.4	65.4 ± 29.7	73.2 ± 31.5[c]
Alpha-amino nitrogen	S	5.58 ± 2.20	4.82 ± 1.61	6.90 ± 2.67
(mg · dL⁻¹)	T	7.72 ± 2.33	6.51 ± 1.13	6.06 ± 2.07
Fetal liver				
Glycogen	S	158.8 ± 28.3	136.4 ± 33.0	109.4 ± 31.9[a]
(μmol · g⁻¹)	T	150.0 ± 65.8	136.8 ± 43.6	124.7 ± 56.4
Triglycerides	S	5.4 ± 0.6	7.5 ± 1.9[a]	7.1 ± 2.9
(μmol · g⁻¹)	T	7.4 ± 1.2[d]	7.6 ± 2.3	8.6 ± 3.2

[a]$p < .05$. [b]$p < .01$ vs resting level. [c]$p < .01$. [d]$p < .001$ vs corresponding values in the sedentary untrained group. S = sedentary, T = trained.

fluid of T group. It increased concentration of uric acid in the amniotic fluid and reduced the content of glycogen in the fetal liver of S group. Training increased total cholesterol concentration in the amniotic fluid and triglyceride content in the fetal liver.

Discussion

The data obtained clearly show that training during pregnancy is not detrimental for the fetus. Therefore, it is not clear why some other investigators employing similar or less intensive training regimes found impaired fetal development (Bonds & Delivoria-Papadopoulos, 1985; Górski, 1985; Mottola et al., 1983). Our study is the first demonstration of the effect of mother's exercise on the amniotic fluid composition. It shows that it is affected only by exercise till exhaustion. The reduction of glucose concentration and an elevation of urea level in T group may be ascribed to longer duration of exercise in T than in S group. On the other hand, the concentration of uric acid increased only in S group, and it may be linked to its elevation in the maternal blood, that occurred only in this group.

The elevation of cholesterol concentration in the amniotic fluid and triglyceride level in the fetal liver in the trained group is difficult to explain. The reduction of glycogen content in the fetal liver during exercise in S group occurred later than it was described previously (Górski, 1983). Interestingly, only insignificant mobilization of glycogen from the liver took place in the T group, despite the prolonged time of exercise. It indicates that training during pregnancy affects metabolism of that substrate in the fetal liver.

References

Bonds, D.R., & Delivoria-Papadopoulos, U. (1985). Exercise during pregnancy—potential fetal and placental metabolic effects. *Ann. Clin. Lab. Sci., 15*, 91-99.

Górski, J. (1985). Exercise during pregnancy: Maternal and fetal responses. A brief review. *Med. Sci. Sports Exerc., 17*, 407-416.

Górski, J. (1983). Effect of exercise on metabolism of energy substrates in pregnant mother and her fetus in the rat. In H.G. Knuttgen, J.A. Vogel, & J. Poortmans (Eds.), *Biochemistry of exercise*. Champaign, IL, Human Kinetics, 229-233.

Mottola, M., Bagnall, K.M., & McFadden, K.D. (1983). The effects of maternal exercise on developing rat fetuses. *Brit. J. Sports Med., 17*, 117-121.

Direct Oxidation of L-Lactate by Mitochondria Isolated From Different Tissues

A. Szczęsna-Kaczmarek

Department of Bioenergetics, Jędrzej Śniadecki Academy of Physical Education, Gdańsk, Poland

This paper describes an unknown until now but general feature of isolated mitochondria—their capability to use L-lactate as a substrate for direct oxidation, coupled to ATP synthesis. It is shown that mitochondria isolated from skeletal muscle, heart, brain, liver, and kidney of the rat, oxidized L-lactate in medium supplemented with external NAD.

Materials and Methods

Mitochondria were isolated from skeletal muscle, liver, brain, kidney, and heart of rats by a method described by Loewenstein et al. (1970). Oxygen uptake was measured at 22 °C with Clark oxygen electrode. The respiratory medium of pH 7.0 contained in a 2-ml volume: 50 mM Trizma-HCl, 40 mM KCl, 5 mM phosphate buffer, 2 mM EDTA, and 0.2% BSA.

Results and Discussion

Oxygen electrode traces obtained with mitochondria from the rat skeletal muscle did not oxidize pyruvate in the absence of malate, whereas in the presence of NAD they were active in mediating oxidation of L-lactate coupled to phosphorylation of ADP.
It has been found that:

1. Among 14 preparations of the rat skeletal muscle mitochondria coupled L-lactate oxidation was demonstrated in 11 cases. The respiratory rate under the state 3 condition varied between 22.5 na O_2 • min^{-1} • mg of $protein^{-1}$ and 82.5 na O_2 • min^{-1} • mg of $protein^{-1}$. The ADP to O ratio varied from 1.27 to 2.27. Respiratory control index (RCI) was between 1.33 to 2.76.

2. In 9 preparations of the rat liver mitochondria in 8 cases coupled L-lactate oxidation was noted. The rate of state 3 respiration ranged from 12 to 35 na O_2 • min^{-1} • mg of $protein^{-1}$. The ADP to O ratio was from 1.3 to 2.1, and RCI from 1.3 to 2.5.

3. Nine preparations of the rat brain mitochondria were active in mediating coupled L-lactate oxidation. The respiratory rate measured during state 3 respiration was between 23 and 60 na O_2 • min^{-1} • mg of $protein^{-1}$. The ratio of ADP to O varied from 1.6 to 2.3, RCI was between 2.28 and 2.7.

4. In 9 preparations of the rat heart mitochondria only 1 did not show coupled L-lactate oxidation. The state 3 ranged from 23 to 42 na O_2 • min^{-1} • mg of $protein^{-1}$. RCI was from 1.14 to 4.0, and ADP to O was from 1.27 to 2.6.

5. All 3 preparations of rat kidney mitochondria were active in L-lactate oxidation. The state 3 rate varied from 25 to 66 na O_2 • min^{-1} • mg of protein^{-1}. The ratio of ADP to O varied from 1.5 to 2.46, and RCI from 1.75 to 2.75.

The oxidation of L-lactate by mitochondria isolated from the rat skeletal muscle and from the liver, kidney, brain, and heart was inhibited by oxamic acid. The similar inhibitory effects obtained with alpha-cyano-3-hydroksyxinnamate, rotenone, malonate, and arsenite indicate participation of the outer mitochondrial membrane LDH, a part of Krebs Cycle and electron transport chain in this oxidation.

Acknowledgments

This work was supported by the grant CPBP 04-01-1-07 from the Polish Academy of Sciences.

Reference

Loewenstein, J., Scholte, H.R., & Wit Peeters, E.M. (1970). A rapid and simple procedure to deplete rat-liver mitochondria of lysosomal activity. *Biochim. Biophys. Acta, 223*, 432-436.

Human Skeletal Muscle Mitochondria: Reevaluation of the Role of the Outer Mitochondrial Membrane in L-Lactate Oxidation

J. Popinigis, A. Szczęsna-Kaczmarek, D. Litwińska, J. Antosiewicz, and K. Krajka

Department of Bioenergetics, Jędrzej Śniadecki Academy of Physical Education and Department of Surgery, School of Medicine, Gdańsk, Poland

Current textbooks do not list L-lactate among substrates which are directly oxidized by mitochondria. Here, and in the accompanying report (Szczęsna-Kaczmarek) we would like to present our experimental data which indicate that mitochondria isolated from human skeletal muscle, as well as those isolated from different rat tissues directly oxidize L-lactate.

Materials and Methods

Muscle samples (mainly from gastrocnemius) were obtained from patients undergoing shank orthopedic amputation. The method employed for the isolation of mitochondria was the same as used earlier for the rat skeletal muscles (Szczęsna-Kaczmarek et al., 1984). Respiration of mitochondria was measured at 20 °C with the Clark-oxygen electrode. The medium (vol 2 ml, pH 7.0) contained 0.2 M sucrose, 50 mM Trizma chloride, 15 mM KCl, 5 mM potassium phosphate, 2 mM EDTA, and 0.2% BSA.

Results

Mitochondria isolated from normal human skeletal muscle mediated direct oxidation of L-lactate. The oxidation was coupled to ADP phosphorylation with ADP to O ratio = 2.47, and was dependent on the presence of external NAD. It can be seen that under the state 3 condition the rate of this respiration reached a value corresponding to 80% of the rate of the state 3 glutamate plus malate oxidation. This NAD-dependent L-lactate oxidation was not found in mitochondrial preparations obtained from skeletal muscle of patients with arteriosclerosis. However, in these cases, the coupled L-lactate oxidation appeared again, or was improved after introducing the dialysed cytoplasmic fraction.

Mitochondria from human skeletal muscle, supplemented with muscle cytoplasm, mediated also a rotenone and antimycin A-insensitive L-lactate oxidation. However, the activity of this ''external pathway''—dependent respiration—was relatively low.

Discussion

This paper demonstrates for the first time that mitochondria isolated from human skeletal muscle mediate a direct and very active oxidation of L-lactate, coupled to ADP phosphorylation. This physiological mechanism was found to be lost or impaired in some diseases, presumably because of decreased binding capacity of the outer mitochondrial membrane to LDH. Human skeletal muscle mitochondria oxidize L-lactate also by a so-called "external pathway" as described previously (Szczęsna-Kaczmarek et al., 1984), but low activity of this pathway does not support our earlier predictions.

Acknowledgments

This work was supported by grant CPBP 04-01-1-07 from the Polish Academy of Sciences.

References

Szczęsna-Kaczmarek, A. (this volume). *Direct oxidation of L-lactate by mitochondria isolated from different tissues.*

Szczęsna-Kaczmarek, A., Litwińska, D., & Popinigis, J. (1984). Oxidation of NADH via an external pathway in skeletal muscle mitochondria and its possible role in the repayment of lactacid oxygen debt. *Int. J. Biochem.,* **16**, 1231-1235.

Effects of Acute Exercise on Insulin Sensitivity Estimated by the Euglycemic Insulin Clamp Technique

Y. Sato, H. Ohno, K. Yamanouchi, S. Hayamizu, C. Yamamoto, and Y. Oshida

Research Center of Health, Physical Fitness and Sports, Nagoya University, Nagoya; First Department of Physiology, Asahikawa Medical College, Asahikawa; and First Department of Internal Medicine, Aichi Medical University, Nagakute, Japan

It has been shown that the euglycemic insulin clamp technique (IC) offers a reliable method for estimating tissue sensitivity to exogenous insulin (DeFronzo et al., 1979). Evidence has been published that physical training increases tissue sensitivity to insulin in proportion to the improvement in physical fitness. We have recently demonstrated that glucose metabolism, determined by IC, directly correlates with maximal oxygen consumption ($\dot{V}O_2max$) ($r = .7269$, $p < .001$), and therefore IC provides a sensitive estimate of training effects (Sato et al., 1984, 1986). The aim of this study was to investigate the influence of each exercise during daily training upon the assessment of long-term training effects. Then, time relationships of insulin sensitivity following acute exercise were examined by IC.

Subjects and Methods

Eleven healthy male volunteers, 19 to 20 years of age, were involved in this study. Six of them were assigned to M group with exercise on a treadmill at a moderate load (40-50% $\dot{V}O_2max$) and the remaining five who performed severe exercise (60-70% $\dot{V}O_2max$) on a bicycle ergometer to S group. All the subjects were examined by IC 120 min before exercise and then immediately, 24, and 72 hours after its termination.

Sensitivity to the in vivo action of insulin was determined with the euglycemic insulin clamp technique as described previously (Sato et al., 1984, 1986). After an overnight fast, a priming (80 mU per square meter of body surface per minute for 10 min) and a continuous infusion (40 mU for 110 min) of crystalline, porcine insulin (Novo Industri A/S, Denmark) was administered for a total of 120 min to obtain a plateau of constant physiologic hyperinsulinemia. The plasma glucose level was maintained at basal preinfusion levels by determination of the plasma glucose concentration every 5 min and the periodic adjustments of the rate of glucose solution infusion. Under such steady-state conditions of constant euglycemia, the whole amount of glucose infused (glucose metabolism) is taken by cells, and thus serves as a measure of the whole body sensitivity to insulin. Urinary catecholamine concentrations were determined by HPLC method.

Results

Urinary catecholamine concentrations in the S group increased ($p < .05$) immediately after exercise, while those in the M group did not show significant changes. Glucose metabolism in the M group at the 4 consecutive time points were 5.53 ± 0.59, 5.71 ± 0.47, 6.61 ± 0.60, and 5.59 ± 0.64 mg • kg^{-1} • min^{-1}. The corresponding values for the S group were 6.55 ± 0.61, 6.02 ± 0.36, 8.21 ± 0.94 ($p < .05$) and 8.32 ± 0.88 ($p < .05$) mg • kg^{-1} • min^{-1}, respectively.

Discussion

Acute exercise has been shown to improve glucose uptake for several hours after exercise, both in humans and in rats. Recently Devlin and Horton (1985) found that an acute high-intensity exercise (85% $\dot{V}O_2$max) significantly increases the insulin-stimulated rates of total glucose disposal in obese subjects for at least 12 to 14 hours. Increases in glucose disposal were also observed in lean subjects, but they did not reach statistical significance, possibly because of the relatively small sample size. The major effect of prior exercise was to increase nonoxidative glucose disposal and glucose oxidation.

Strenuous exercise results in increased levels of circulating catecholamines. Secretion of catecholamines is proportional to the amount of work performed. The potential effect of rising norepinephrine levels on maintenance of metabolic fuel supply is significant because norepinephrine inhibits insulin secretion, while at the same time it stimulates glucagon and growth hormone secretion (Vignati & Cunningham, 1985).

Our present results indicate that insulin sensitivity remains improved for at least 3 days following the exercise at a load of 60 to 70% $\dot{V}O_2$max while exercise at lower loads 40 to 50% $\dot{V}O_2$max, employed in ordinary exercise treatment, fails to induce similar favorable changes in insulin sensitivity. In view of the tendency towards an increase in glucose metabolism 24 hours after exercise, it seems advisable to discontinue training for at least 2 days prior to IC while assessing the effects of a long-term training program.

References

DeFronzo, R.A., Tobin, J.D., & Andres, R. (1979). Glucose clamp technique: A method for quantifying insulin secretion and resistance. *Am. J. Physiol.*, **237**, E214-E223.

Devlin, J.T., & Horton, E.S. (1985). Effects of prior high-intensity exercise on glucose metabolism in normal and insulin-resistant men. *Diabetes,* **34**, 973-979.

Sato, Y., Iguchi, A., & Sakamoto, N. (1984). Biochemical determination of training effects using insulin clamp technique. *Horm. Metab. Res.,* **16**, 483-486.

Sato, Y., Hayamizu, S., Yamamoto, C., Ohkuwa, Y., Yamanouch, K., & Sakamoto, N. (1986). Improved insulin sensitivity in carbohydrate and lipid metabolism after physical training. *Int. J. Sports Med.,* **7**, 307-310.

Vignati, L., & Cunningham, L.N. (1985). Exercise and diabetes. In *Joslin's diabetes mellitus* (12th ed.). Lea and Febiger, Philadelphia, 453-464.

The Effect of Exercise on Lipoprotein Lipase Activity in Skeletal Muscle and Heart of Rats With Thyroid Hormone Deficit or Excess

E.M. Jabłońska, L. Budohoski, and J. Langfort
Department of Applied Physiology, Medical Research Centre, Polish
Academy of Sciences, Warsaw, Poland

Lipoprotein lipase (LPL) is an essential enzyme responsible for hydrolysis of circulating triacylglycerols (TG) which makes fatty acids available for the tissue uptake. Changes in tissue LPL activity occur in response to a variety of situations such as physical exercise, starvation, lactation, etc. (Borensztajn, 1987; Cryer, 1981). However, the effects of hormones on LPL activity remain unclear. There are few data on the effects of thyroid state on this enzyme activity (Kaciuba-Uściłko et al., 1980; Skottova et al., 1983; Wirth et al., 1981). Our aim was to investigate the influence of experimentally modified thyroid hormone level in blood on the exercise-induced changes in the activity of two forms of LPL in the soleus muscle and myocardium.

Material and Methods

Male Wistar rats (200-220 g b.w.) were used. They were divided into three groups. In the PTU group the animals were treated with 0.04% propylthiouracyl (PTU) given in drinking water for 3 weeks ($n = 16$), and in the T_3 group they were injected with triiodothyronine (daily i.p. injections of 75 μgT$_3$/100 g b.w.) ($n = 18$). The C (control) group consisted of 22 intact rats. Each group was divided into two subgroups: sedentary (S) and exercised (Ex). The exercising rats ran on a motor driven treadmill at 20 m $\times$ min^{-1}, 0^0 inclination for 30 min. Before each experiment rats were deprived of food for 18 to 24 h. They were sacrificed by decapitation. Blood was collected for radioimmunoassay determination of thyroxine (T_4) and triiodothyronine (T_3). Soleus muscle and heart were immediately dissected and frozen. Lipoprotein lipase activity (LPLA) was determined by measuring the release of (^{14}C) oleic acid from the emulsion of glycerol-tri (^{14}C) oleate in a medium containing albumin and human serum according to the modified method of Taskinen et al. (1980). The extracellular form of LPL was released from the tissue with heparin, and the intracellular form was measured in the homogenate. LPLA was expressed as μmol of FFA released by 1 g of tissue in 1 h. Statistical analysis was performed using Student's t test.

Results and Conclusion

As shown in Table 1, PTU feeding significantly decreased thyroid hormone level in blood, whereas T_3 treatment increased T_3 and decreased T_4 level. The exercise performed caused no changes in serum concentration of these hormones. As expected, LPLA was altered by modified thyroid hormone level. In PTU-treated rats an increase in the extracellular

Table 1   Serum Concentration of Thyroid Hormones in Sedentary Control (C), Thyroid-Hormone Deficient (PTU), and Triiodothyronine-Treated (T_3) Rats

Hormone concentration (ng $\times$ ml^{-1})	PTU	C	T_3
T_3	0.13 ± 0.02*	0.49 ± 0.05	>100*
T_4	12.60 ± 0.90*	46.40 ± 2.20	27.8 ± 1.20*

*Significantly different from controls, $p < .001$.

and a decrease in the intracellular forms of LPL in the soleus muscle were found. Myocardial LPLA was not affected by PTU treatment. In the rats with T_3 excess the activity of two forms of LPL was decreased in both muscles. A single bout of exercise caused an enhancement of LPL activity (both forms) only in the thyroid-hormone deficient rats. The changes in the tissue LPLA may be due to a direct action of thyroid hormones on this enzyme or to the altered metabolic state of cells (e.g., availability of free fatty acids). An inhibitory effect of free fatty acids on LPLA has been previously reported (Budohoski et al., 1985).

Thyroid hormone deficit is associated with increased skeletal muscle LPL activity, whereas the hormone excess results in reduction of LPL activity both in skeletal and cardiac muscles. Physical exercise causes further enhancement of the enzyme activity (both intra- and extra-cellular forms) in the thyroid-hormone deficient animals.

Acknowledgments

This work was supported by the Polish Central Programme for Basic Research 06.02. III.2.1.

References

Borensztajn, J. (1987). Heart and skeletal muscle lipoprotein lipase. In J. Borensztajn (Ed.), *Lipoprotein lipase*. Evener Publishers, Chicago, 133-148.

Budohoski, L., Kozłowski, S., Kaciuba-Uściłko, H., & Nazar, K. (1985). Free fatty acids: The possible regulators of muscle lipoprotein lipase. *Biochem. Soc. Trans.*, **13**, 129-130.

Cryer, A. (1981). Tissue lipoprotein lipase activity and its action in lipoprotein metabolism. *Int. J. Biochem.*, **13**, 525-541.

Kaciuba-Uściłko, H., Dudley, G.A., & Terjung, R.A. (1980). Influence of thyroid status on skeletal muscle LPL activity and TG uptake. *Am. J. Physiol.*, **238**(Endocrinol. Metab. 1), E518-E523.

Skottova, N., Wallinder, L., & Bengtsson, G. (1983). Activity of lipoprotein lipase in thyroidectomized rats. *Biochim. Biophys. Acta*, **750**, 533-538.

Taskinen, M.R., Nikkila, E.A., Huttunen, J.K., & Hilden, H. (1980). A micromethod for assay of lipoprotein lipase activity in needle biopsy samples of human adipose tissue and skeletal muscle. *Clin. Chim. Acta*, **104**, 107-117.

Wirth, A., Holm, G., Lindsted, G., Lundberg, P.A., & Bjorntorp, P. (1981). Thyroid hormones and lipolysis in physically trained rats. *Metabolism*, **30**(3), 237-241.

The Effects of Acute and Chronic Insulin Deprivation on Skeletal Muscle Metabolism During Contractile Activity in the Diabetic Rat

R.A.J. Challiss, D.J. Hayes, M.J. Brosnan, M. Vranic, and G.K. Radda

Department of Biochemistry, University of Oxford, Oxford, and Department of Pharmacology, University of Leicester, Leicester, U.K.

A complex array of morphological, physiological, and biochemical changes have been documented to occur in skeletal muscle during chronic hypoinsulinemia. A disease state similar to that seen in untreated insulin-dependent diabetes mellitus (IDDM) can be caused by administration of the diabetogenic agent streptozotocin in rats (Rerup, 1970). With this agent, the severity of the resultant disease is dose-related (Ganda et al., 1976) and at low doses (45-65 mg/Kg body wt.) a diabetic state can be produced where plasma glucose is elevated (> 20 mM), plasma insulin is reduced ($> 90\%$), but ketoacidosis is modest. This reduces mortality and allows chronic changes in the diabetic state to be investigated.

Surprisingly little work has been carried out to assess the metabolic consequences of the diabetic state on muscle performance and bioenergetics during exercise (see Wasserman & Vranic, 1986). Until recently, it had generally been accepted that glucose transport into the contracting muscle mass may be compromised during exercise in the insulinopenic state; however, recent experiments have given evidence to suggest that muscle contraction per se is sufficient to increase glucose transport (Nesher et al., 1985; Ploug et al., 1984; Wallberg-Henriksson & Holloszy, 1984). A question not addressed by these in vitro studies is the possibility that glucose transport may be affected by the high concentrations of fatty acids, ketone bodies, and exaggerated increases in counterregulatory hormones seen in vivo in the diabetic state (Wasserman & Vranic, 1986). Furthermore, the consequences of changes in activities of enzymes of the glycolytic and oxidative pathways with respect to contractile performance has not generally been addressed.

In the present study we have assessed the effects of acute (3 days) and chronic (21 days) untreated streptozotocin diabetes on skeletal muscle performance and bioenergetics during contraction. We have used ^{31}P-nuclear magnetic resonance (NMR) spectroscopy to determine changes in muscle metabolites and intracellular pH during isometric muscle contraction in vivo and have attempted to correlate changes in muscle physiological performance and energy status with changes in enzyme activities occurring in muscle of diabetic animals.

Methods

Male Wistar rats (140-160 g) received an intravenous injection of 50 mg/Kg body wt. streptozotocin in 50 mM citrate buffer (pH 4.5). Control animals received an equivalent volume (1 ml/Kg) of citrate buffer only. All animals given streptozotocin developed a marked hyperglycemia and glucosuria within 48 h. Upon diagnosis, rats either received subcutaneous injections of Ultratard insulin (Novo, Copenhagen, Denmark) administered twice-daily to maintain optimal glycemic control, or remained untreated to the period to the time of study.

Four experimental groups were studied: (1) nondiabetic controls (CON); (2) diabetics treated with insulin throughout the experimental period (ITD); (3) diabetics treated with insulin until 72 h before study (IWD); and (4) untreated diabetics (UD). All animals were given free access to food and water and were studied 21 to 22 days after streptozotocin or vehicle administration.

Animals were prepared for study as described previously (Challiss et al., 1986). Isometric contraction of gastrocnemius muscle was caused by sciatic nerve stimulation and tension development was recorded using a force-displacement transducer attached to the distal tendon of the gastrocnemius muscle. A surface coil placed over the medial head of the gastrocnemius muscle was used for ^{31}P-NMR spectrospcopy. NMR experiments were performed at 73.84 MHz in a 4.3 T wide-bore magnet (Challiss et al., 1986). After collection of resting spectra, the sciatic nerve was stimulated at a supramaximal voltage (50 μs pulse-width, 45V) at 1 Hz for 22 min and at 5 Hz for 10 min. The time-resolution of NMR data acquisition was determined by signal to noise considerations and was about 2 min (64 transients, 2 s pulse-delay). After stimulation, recovery was followed for 30 min and the gastrocnemius muscles of the stimulated and contralateral limbs freeze-clamped for subsequent analysis of tissue ATP and total creatine (creatine plus phosphocreatine) to allow quantitation of phosphorus-containing metabolites from ^{31}P-NMR spectra (Challis et al., 1986; Taylor et al., 1983).

Adenine nucleotides, phosphocreatine (PCr) and creatine were determined by the high performance liquid chromatographic method of Harmsen et al. (1982). Insulin was determined in the plasma fraction obtained after centrifugation of a freshly drawn arterial blood sample (Albano et al., 1972). Glucose (Bergmeyer et al., 1973), fatty acids (Okabe et al., 1980), and 3-hydroxybutyrate (Williamson et al., 1962) were determined in deproteinized blood samples. Activities of hexokinase, phosphorylase$_{[a+b]}$, citrate synthase, and 3-hydroxy acyl CoA dehydrogenase in homogenates of gastrocnemius muscle, and pyruvate dehydrogenase (PDH) in isolated skeletal muscle mitochondria (see below), were determined as described previously (Hayes et al., 1985; Shoubridge et al., 1985).

Skeletal muscle mitochondria were isolated from gastrocnemius muscle by the method of Morgan-Hughes et al. (1977). Mitochondria from chronically diabetic animals exhibited high respiratory rates in the presence of ADP, but in the absence of exogenously added substrates. To obtain mitochondria dependent on exogenous substrates, the mitochondrial pellet obtained from gastrocnemius muscle of CON, IWD, or UD donor animals was initially suspended in 10 ml of respiration medium (Morgan-Hughes et al., 1977) containing 50 μmol ADP. After incubation at 25 °C for 10 min a further 15 ml of respiration medium was added and the mitochondria isolated by centrifugation (8000 g, 15 min, 4 °C).

Where appropriate, one-way analysis of variance and multiple comparisons by testing linear functions (or by Bonferroni t tests) were carried out using the SAS statistical package (SAS Institute, Cary, NC, USA). In addition, Student's t test has been applied. All results are reported as means $\pm$ SE and statistical significance between mean values was defined as $p < .05$.

Results and Discussion

Table 1 gives some general characteristics of the four experimental groups. Untreated streptozotocin-diabetic rats were hypoinsulinemic and hyperglycemic, plasma fatty acid and ketone body concentrations were increased 2 to 3 fold; thus, the derangement of lipid metabolism seen in this diabetic model may be considered modest compared to changes seen in diabetes induced using higher doses of streptozotocin or alloxan (Ganda et al.,

Table 1   Body Weights and Plasma Insulin, Glucose, Fatty Acids and 3-Hydroxy-butyrate Concentrations in Insulin-Treated, Insulin-Withdrawn, and Untreated Diabetic Rats

	Control	Insulin-treated	Insulin-withdrawn	Untreated
Period of diabetes (days)	0	21 ± 1	22 ± 1	21 ± 1
Period without insulin (days)	—	0	3	21
Body wt. gain (g/day)	5.0 ± 0.2	3.4 ± 0.3	3.2 ± 0.4	0.9 ± 0.3
Plasma concentrations				
Insulin (μU/ml)	20.6 ± 4.2	N.D.	3.4 ± 0.7	2.8 ± 0.4
Glucose (mM)	8.3 ± 0.6	6.9 ± 1.0	22.8 ± 1.3	24.4 ± 1.8
Fatty acids (mM)	0.26 ± 0.02	N.D.	0.57 ± 0.07	0.71 ± 0.06
3-hydroxybutyrate (mM)	0.09 ± 0.03	N.D.	0.33 ± 0.09	0.28 ± 0.10

Note. Results are given as means ± *SE* for six animals in each experimental group. N.D. = not determined.

1976). Withdrawal of insulin treatment from diabetic rats caused a rapid re-onset of the diabetic state, such that 72 h after insulin withdrawal, plasma insulin and metabolite levels were identical to those measured in untreated diabetic animals.

Untreated streptozotocin diabetes for 3 weeks resulted in a significant 38% decrease in hexokinase activity in gastrocnemius muscle (Table 2), a finding consistent with that of others (Chen & Ianuzzo, 1982). However, no change in phosphorylase activity was observed. Small, statistically insignificant changes in citrate synthase and 3-hydroxyacyl CoA dehydrogenase activities were seen in chronic diabetes consistent with, but smaller than, the changes reported by Chen and Ianuzzo (1982). Insulin-treatment of diabetic animals prevented changes in any of the enzyme activities measured and withdrawal of insulin for 72 h caused no significant changes in enzyme activities.

Respiratory activities for mitochondria isolated from gastrocnemius muscles of insulin-withdrawn and untreated diabetics and for control animals are shown in Table 3. Conflicting results for the effects of diabetes on mitochondrial function and metabolism have been reported in the literature (see Rogers et al., 1986 for references and discussion). We noted that mitochondria isolated from skeletal muscle of untreated diabetic animals exhibited high rates of oxygen consumption in the presence of ADP, but in the absence of exogenously added substrates, suggesting that endogenous oxidative substrates were being utilized. To ensure measurement of exogenous substrate-dependent respiratory rates, we pre-incubated isolated mitochondria (all experimental groups) with excess ADP, to deplete endogenous substrate, prior to performing the assays presented in Table 3. Under these conditions it is clear that respiratory activities in the presence of NAD-linked substrates are significantly decreased in mitochondria from skeletal muscle of untreated diabetic rats. Furthermore, a significant decrease of 26% was observed when succinate was added as sole substrate. In contrast, ascorbate/TMPD respiratory rates were similar for all mitochondrial preparations.

Table 2   Maximal Activities of Hexokinasea, Phosphorylase, Citrate Synthase and 3-Hydroxyacyl CoA Dehydrogenase in Gastrocnemius Muscle of Insulin-Treated, Insulin-Withdrawn and Untreated Diabetic Rats

	Control	Insulin-treated	Insulin-withdrawn	Untreated
Hexokinase	0.96 ± 0.10	0.91 ± 0.11	0.89 ± 0.19	0.59 ± 0.13*
Phosphorylase	38.9 ± 3.1	38.4 ± 2.6	38.7 ± 3.4	36.0 ± 2.7
Citrate synthase	18.0 ± 3.1	19.7 ± 2.4	17.1 ± 2.7	15.2 ± 2.2
3-Hydroxyacyl CoA DH	3.4 ± 0.4	3.9 ± 0.7	3.9 ± 0.4	4.7 ± 0.5

Note. Results are given as means ± SE for at least 5 determinations in each experimental group. *$p < .05$ (unpaired Student's t test) for untreated diabetic versus nondiabetic control. Maximal activity (μmol • min^{-1} per g of tissue at 25 °C).

Table 3   Respiratory and Enzyme Activities in Mitochondria Isolated From Gastrocnemius Muscles of Insulin-Treated, Insulin-Withdrawn, and Untreated Diabetic Rats

	Control	Insulin-withdrawn	Untreated
5 mM pyruvate + 2.5 mM L-malate	172 ± 18	156 ± 21	121 ± 13*
5 mM glutamate + 2.5 mM L-malate	164 ± 13	137 ± 24	110 ± 16*
10 mM DL-succinate + 10 μM rotenone	241 ± 11	197 ± 21	178 ± 25*
2 mM L-ascorbate + 50 μM TMPD	444 ± 36	469 ± 32	502 ± 47
Pyruvate dehydrogenase[a]	118 ± 21	130 ± 17	102 ± 26

Note. 2-3 gastrocnemius muscles were combined for each preparation of mitochondria. Results are given as means ± SE for at least 5 mitochondrial preparations for each experimental group. Respiratory control ratios (R.C.R.) were >5 for NAD-linked substrates and >3 for succinate. There were no differences in R.C.R.s between experimental groups. Pyruvate dehydrogenase (PDH) was determined in isolated mitochondria after 10 min pre-incubation with 0.1 mM Ca^{++} and 1.0 mM Mg^{++} to fully activate PDH (see Hayes et al., 1986). *$p < .05$ (Students unpaired t test) for untreated diabetic versus nondiabetic control groups. TMPD - tetramethylphenylaminediamine. Respiratory activities (natoms 0 • min^{-1} per mg mitochondrial protein at 30 °C). [a]Maximal enzyme activity (mmol • min^{-1} per mg mitochondrial protein at 30 °C).

Withdrawal of insulin treatment from diabetic rats for 72 h before mitochondrial preparation caused 10 to 15% decreases in pyruvate-, glutamate-, and succinate-linked respiratory rates; however, none of these effects were statistically significantly different from control values. PDH activity was measured in isolated mitochondria after enzymic activation by pre-incubation with Ca^{++} and Mg^{++}; no differences in total activity were found, consistent with the results of other workers (Fuller & Randle, 1984). Therefore, it is likely that the decreased rate of pyruvate oxidation measured in isolated diabetic mitochondria is due to a reversible modification of PDH activity which is maintained through the mitochondrial isolation procedure. It is well established that PDH activity is decreased in heart and skeletal muscle in diabetes by increased phosphorylation of the enzyme; this is brought about, at least in part, by an increase in PDH kinase activity (Fuller & Randle, 1984).

Initial twitch-tension was similar for insulin-treated, insulin-withdrawn and chronically diabetic rats: 1.53 ± 0.08 (6); 1.60 ± 0.07 (6); and 1.38 ± 0.16 (6) g/g body wt. for ITD, IWD, and UD animals, respectively. Although tension development by gastrocnemius muscle of chronically diabetic rats tended to decline through the period of stimulation at 1 Hz compared to the insulin-treated group, significant differences were not observed until the stimulation frequency was increased to 5 Hz. At the end of the period of stimulation at 5 Hz, gastrocnemius muscle twitch-tension was 0.57 ± 0.10 (6) and 1.03 ± 0.08 (6) g/g body wt. for chronically diabetic and insulin-treated diabetic animals, respectively ($p < .01$). In contrast, muscle performance for 72 h insulin-withdrawn diabetic rats was similar to that of the insulin-treated group and twitch-tension was significantly higher in this group compared to the chronically diabetic group ($p < .05$).

Data obtained by ^{31}P-NMR spectroscopy are presented in Table 4. During gastrocnemius muscle stimulation at 1 Hz, PCr concentration and intracellular pH were significantly lower (and P_i concentration higher) in chronically diabetic animals compared to either insulin-treated or nondiabetic controls. Thus, in chronic diabetes muscle performance (twitch-tension) at 1 Hz was maintained with increased PCr utilization and a lower intracellular pH, suggesting a greater dependence on glycolytic ATP production.

In contrast, muscle stimulation at 5 Hz exacerbated relative intracellular acidosis in chronically diabetic animals; PCr and P_i concentrations were similar to those observed in muscle of control and insulin-treated diabetic rats; but twitch-tension was reduced by 35 to 45% throughout this period of stimulation in the chronically diabetic group. Therefore, in chronic diabetes muscle performance at 5 Hz was compromised, and the results presented here are consistent with the hypothesis that glycolytic mechanisms for ATP production are inadequate at this stimulation intensity, with the exaggerated intracellular acidosis being a possible important contributory factor.

Previous studies have shown that exercise increases the proportion of PDH in the active form in skeletal muscle and that this activation is attenuated in the diabetic state (Hagg et al., 1976; Hennig et al., 1975). With respect to this, it is important to note that withdrawal of insulin for 72 h from diabetic rats, which caused complete reversal of plasma insulin and metabolite levels to the diabetic state, did not significantly affect contractile performance or muscle bioenergetics in the present study; (Table 4); thus, chronic hypoinsulinaemia is necessary to cause these alterations in skeletal muscle.

Acknowledgments

We thank the British Heart Foundation and the Medical Research Council for financial support. M. Vranic was a Visiting Research Fellow of Merton College Oxford and acknowledges financial support from the Medical Research Council of Canada. Statistical analysis was performed by Debbie Bilinski (Department of Physiology, Toronto University) and we thank Melanie Burnett (Diabetes Research Laboratories, Radcliffe Infirmary, Oxford) for assaying insulin.

References

Albano, J.D.M., Edkins, R.P., Maritz, G., & Turner, R.C. (1972). A sensitive, precise radioimmunoassay of serum insulin relying on charcoal separation of bound and free moieties. *Acta Endocrinol. (Copenh.), 70,* 487-497.

Table 4   Changes in Phosphocreatine and Inorganic Phosphate Concentrations and Intracellular pH in Gastrocnemius Muscle of Insulin-Treated (ITD), Insulin-Withdrawn (IWD), and Untreated (UD) Diabetic Rats and Nondiabetic Controls (CON) at Rest, During Muscle Stimulation at 1 and 5 Hz and After Recovery.

Time of stimulation		Concentration (μmol/g of tissue)		
		PCr	P_i	pH_i
Rest	CON	26.4 $\pm$ 0.6	2.7 $\pm$ 0.3	7.04 $\pm$ 0.03
	ITD	26.2 $\pm$ 0.5	2.9 $\pm$ 0.5	7.02 $\pm$ 0.02
	IWD	26.1 $\pm$ 0.6	2.7 $\pm$ 0.2	6.99 $\pm$ 0.02
	UD	25.1 $\pm$ 0.7	3.5 $\pm$ 0.6	6.94 $\pm$ 0.03[ab]
10 min	CON	19.2 $\pm$ 1.4	10.1 $\pm$ 0.5	6.94 $\pm$ 0.02
1 Hz	ITD	18.9 $\pm$ 0.9	10.1 $\pm$ 0.6	6.95 $\pm$ 0.01
	IWD	17.4 $\pm$ 0.6	10.9 $\pm$ 0.8	6.96 $\pm$ 0.02
	UD	15.1 $\pm$ 0.9[ab]	13.2 $\pm$ 0.8[ab]	6.86 $\pm$ 0.03[bc]
20 min	CON	19.6 $\pm$ 1.5	9.8 $\pm$ 0.5	6.96 $\pm$ 0.01
1 Hz	ITD	19.4 $\pm$ 0.9	9.6 $\pm$ 0.5	6.96 $\pm$ 0.01
	IWD	18.0 $\pm$ 0.9	10.4 $\pm$ 0.6	6.97 $\pm$ 0.02
	UD	15.3 $\pm$ 0.9[ab]	13.0 $\pm$ 0.8[abc]	6.86 $\pm$ 0.02[abc]
5 min	CON	8.2 $\pm$ 1.1	21.6 $\pm$ 1.9	6.75 $\pm$ 0.03
5 Hz	ITD	7.7 $\pm$ 1.0	21.6 $\pm$ 1.4	6.79 $\pm$ 0.02
	IWD	6.4 $\pm$ 0.7	22.9 $\pm$ 1.0	6.80 $\pm$ 0.03
	UD	6.2 $\pm$ 0.6	21.8 $\pm$ 1.4	6.56 $\pm$ 0.05[abc]
10 min	CON	8.6 $\pm$ 1.1	21.0 $\pm$ 1.3	6.89 $\pm$ 0.02
5 Hz	ITD	8.1 $\pm$ 0.8	21.0 $\pm$ 1.3	6.89 $\pm$ 0.02
	IWD	8.5 $\pm$ 1.1	20.7 $\pm$ 0.9	6.89 $\pm$ 0.03
	UD	7.4 $\pm$ 0.6	20.4 $\pm$ 1.2	6.72 $\pm$ 0.03[abc]
Recovery	CON	25.7 $\pm$ 0.7	2.4 $\pm$ 0.2	7.01 $\pm$ 0.02
	ITD	25.8 $\pm$ 0.6	2.2 $\pm$ 0.4	6.98 $\pm$ 0.02
	IWD	25.1 $\pm$ 0.8	2.7 $\pm$ 0.3	6.98 $\pm$ 0.03
	UD	23.9 $\pm$ 1.3	2.5 $\pm$ 0.5	6.93 $\pm$ 0.03

Note. ^{31}P-NMR experiments were performed as described in the methods section. Values obtained from NMR spectra (Taylor et al., 1983) are presented as means $\pm$ SE for six experiments in each group. Statistical significance (Student's t test, for unpaired observations) is indicated as $^ap < .05$, UD versus CON; $^bp < .05$, UD versus ITD; $^cp < .05$, UD versus IWD.

Bergmeyer, H.-U, Bernt, E., Schmidt, F., & Stork, H. (1973). In Bergmeyer (Ed.), *Methods of enzymatic analysis.* Academic Press, New York, 1196-1201.

Challiss, R.A.J., Hayes, D.J., Petty, P.F.H., & Radda, G.K. (1986). An investigation of arterial insufficiency in rat hindlimb: A combined ^{31}P-NMR and bloodflow study. *Biochem. J., 236,* 461-467.

Chen, V., & Ianuzzo, C.D. (1982). Metabolic alterations in skeletal muscle of chronically streptozotocin-diabetic rates. *Arch. Biochem. Biophys., 217,* 131-138.

Fuller, S.J., & Randle, P.J. (1984). Reversible phosphorylation of pyruvate dehydrogenase in rat skeletal muscle mitochondria. *Biochem. J., 219,* 635-646.

Ganda, O.P., Rossini, A.A., & Like, A.A. (1976). Studies on streptozotocin diabetes. *Diabetes*, **25**, 595-603.

Hagg, S.A., Taylor, S.I., & Ruderman, N.B. (1976). Glucose metabolism in perfused skeletal muscle: Pyruvate dehydrogenase activity in starvation, diabetes and exercise. *Biochem. J.*, **158**, 203-210.

Harmsen, E., DeTombe, P.P., & DeJong, J.W. (1982). Simultaneous determination of myocardial adenine nucleotides and cretine phosphate by high performance liquid chromatography. *J. Chromatogr.*, **230**, 131-136.

Hayes, D.J., Challiss, R.A.J., & Radda, G.K. (1986). An investigation of arterial insufficiency in rat hindlimb: An enzymic, mitochondrial and histological study. *Biochem. J.*, **236**, 469-473.

Hennig, G., Loffler, G., & Wieland, O.H. (1975). Active and inactive forms of pyruvate dehydrogenase in skeletal muscle as related to the metabolic and functional state of the muscle cell. *FEBS Lett.*, **59**, 142-145.

Morgan-Hughes, J.A., Dareniza, P., Kahn, S.N., Landon, D.N., Sherratt, J.M., Land, J.M., & Clark, J.B. (1977). A mitochondrial myopathy characterized by a deficiency in reducible cytochrome$_b$. *Brain*, **100**, 27-46.

Nesher, R., Karl, I.E., & Kipnis, D.M. (1985). Dissociation of effects of insulin and contraction on glucose transport in rat epitrochlearis muscle. *Am. J. Physiol.*, **249**, C226-C232.

Okabe, H., Uji, Y., Nagashima, K., & Noma, A. (1980). Enzymic determination of free fatty acids in serum. *Clin. Chem.*, **26**, 1540-1543.

Ploug, T., Galbo, H., & Richter, E.A. (1984). Increased muscle glucose uptake during contractions: No need for insulin. *Am. J. Physiol.*, **247**, E726-E731.

Rerup, C.C. (1970). Drugs producing diabetes through damage of the insulin secreting cells. *Pharmacol. Rev.*, **22**, 485-518.

Rogers, K.S., Friend, W.H., & Higgins, E.S. (1986). Metabolic and mitochondrial disturbances in streptozotocin-treated Sprague-Dawley and Sherman rats. *Proc. Soc. Exp. Biol. Med.*, **182**, 167-175.

Shoubridge, E.A., Challiss, R.A.J., Hayes, D.J., & Radda, G.K. (1985). Biochemical adaptation in the skeletal muscle of rats depleted of creatine with the substrate analogue β-guanidinopropionic acid. *Biochem. J.*, **232**, 125-131.

Taylor, D.J., Bore, P.J., Styles, P., Gadian, D.G., & Radda, G.K. (1983). Bioenergetics of human muscle: A ^{31}P-NMR study. *Mol. Biol. Med.*, **1**, 77-94.

Wallberg-Henriksson, H., & Holloszy, J.O. (1984). Contractile activity increases glucose uptake by muscle in severely diabetic rats. *J. Appl. Physiol.*, **57**, 1045-1049.

Wasserman, D.H., & Vranic, M. (1986). Interaction between insulin and counterregulatory hormones in control of substrate utilization in health and diabetes during exercise. *Diabetes/Metabolism Rev.*, **1**, 359-384.

Williamson, D.H., Mellanby, J., & Krebs, H.A. (1962). Enzymatic determination of D(−) β-hydroxybutyric acid and acetoacetic acid in blood. *Biochem. J.*, **82**, 90-96.

The Effect of Exercise of Different Characteristics on Red and White Muscle Sensitivity to Insulin

J. Langfort, L. Budohoski, and E.A. Newsholme

Department of Applied Physiology, Medical Research Centre, Polish Academy of Sciences, Warsaw, Poland and Department of Biochemistry, University of Oxford, Oxford, U.K.

Physical activity is known to improve insulin sensitivity, as reflected by a smaller increase in the plasma insulin concentration in response to a glucose load and unchanged or improved glucose tolerance. As a possible mechanism of this effect an increased sensitivity of muscles to insulin has been suggested. The aim of the present study was to find out whether the effect of exercise on the muscle insulin sensitivity depends on muscle fiber composition. For this purpose insulin sensitivity of the soleus (containing mainly ST fibers) and epitrochlearis m. (containing mainly FT glycolytic fibers) was examined in vitro in rats subjected to exercise of various characteristics.

Male Wistar rats (160-180 g) were used for this study. They were randomly selected into three groups: (1) sedentary controls, (2) exercised for 60 min at moderate intensity (treadmill run at 20 m $\times$ min^{-1}, 0° incl.), and (3) subjected to "sprint" exercise (six repetitions of a 10 s run at 43 m $\times$ min^{-1} with 50 s resting intervals between them). Animals from the exercising groups were decapitated 0.25, 2, or 24 h after the runs and epitrochlearis (ET) and soleus (S) m. were rapidly dissected. Each time 7 rats were used. Muscle strips were incubated in Krebs-Ringer bicarbonate buffer containing 1.5% deffated albumin, 5.5 mM glucose, U-^{14}C glucose (0.25 μCi $\times$ ml^{-1}) and insulin in concentration varying from 1 to 10000 μU $\times$ ml^{-1}. Muscle insulin sensitivity was expressed as the concentration of insulin required to produce the half-maximum stimulation of lactate formation or glycogen synthesis. This was calculated based on the computer log-logit transformation of the data. In some rats from each group, muscle glycogen content in both muscles was measured.

Glycogen content both in S and ET m. was depleted more after "sprint" than endurance exercise. In the latter case it returned to the resting level within 2 h. Sensitivity of lactate production to insulin in ET m. was significantly enhanced both after "sprint" and after endurance exercise (Table 1). Sensitivity of lactate production to insulin in the S m. was increased only after endurance exercise. Sensitivity of glycogen synthesis to insulin was found to be increased in ET m. only 0.25 h after "sprint" exercise and in S m. 24 h after endurance exercise. The basal (insulin unstimulated) rate of glycogen synthesis increased significantly after both exercise types in ET m., while in S m. it was elevated only after endurance exercise.

In conclusion, this study showed that the insulin sensitivity of lactate formation and glycogen synthesis in epitrochlearis and soleus muscles are similar at rest. In the fast-twitch muscle (ET) both "sprint" and endurance exercise increased sensitivity of lactate formation, while in slow-twitch muscle (S) only endurance exercise exerted this effect. Changes in glycogen synthesis sensitivity to insulin were less pronounced; however, a transient increase occurred in the fast-twitch muscle shortly after "sprint" exercise and in the slow-twitch muscle in the latter period (24 h) following endurance exercise.

Table 1   Insulin concentration (μU · ml^{-1}) Inducing the Half-Maximal Stimulation of Lactate Formation or Glycogen Synthesis in Slow-Twitch (Soleus) and Fast-Twitch (Epitrochlearis) Muscles in Resting and Exercising Rats

	Muscle	Sedentary controls	Time after endurance exercise (h)			Time after sprint exercise (h)		
			0.25	2	24	0.25	2	24
Lactate formation	Soleus	122.46 ±13.40	17.10* ±12.32	38.11* ±13.42	124.16 ±64.00	211.84 ±55.46	165.19 ±35.71	135.92 ±26.63
	Epitrochlearis	120.50 ±17.22	71.28* ±21.61	63.53* ±15.17	106.16 ±35.41	58.88* ±14.23	30.13 ± 9.77	92.46 ±21.82
Glycogen synthesis	Soleus	81.85 ± 9.72	120.50 ±23.04	58.08 ±46.05	43.65* ±14.02	250.19 ±69.44	153.11 ±64.66	98.17 ±21.22
	Epitrochlearis	97.05 ±11.84	97.38 ±22.19	101.39 ±16.37	87.07 ±15.49	38.90* ± 5.66	76.03 ± 6.86	83.17 ±14.77

Note. Mean ± S.E.M. *Significant differences in comparison with sedentary controls.

Effects of Cold Swimming on Serum Lipids, HDL Lipoproteins, and Lecithin: Cholesterol Acyltransferase Activity in Male and Female Rats

C. Tsopanakis, E. Sgourakis, and C. Tesserommatis

Experimental Physiology and Pharmacology Departments, Athens University Medical School and Exercise Biochemistry Laboratory, Hellenic Sports Research Institute, Athens, Greece

Stress has been reported to result in changes of serum cholesterol and can be a risk factor for coronary heart disease (CHD). Our purpose was to investigate the effects of cold stress on parameters of lipid metabolism, namely serum cholesterol (TC), triglycerides (TG), HDL-C, free fatty acids (FFA), and activity of the enzyme lecithin—cholesterol acyltransferase (LCAT)—that plays a key role in HDL-C metabolism.

Subjects were 40 female and 46 male Wistar rats (age 40 ± 5 days) divided into the following groups: (1) Female: A_1 ($n = 10$), A_2 ($n = 10$), and B ($n = 20$). Groups $A_{1,2}$ were subjected to everyday cold swimming stress (5 °C for 10 min) for 10 and 20 days respectively: Group B was used as controls. (2) Male: C_1 ($n = 10$), C_2 ($n = 10$), C_3 ($n = 10$), and D ($n = 16$). Groups $C_{1,2,3}$ received the same as above treatment for 20, 40, and 60 days, respectively, while D was used as controls. Serum cholesterol levels showed a statistically significant decrease from 10 days in female rats ($p < .01$), while in males the decrease appeared from 40 days ($p < .001$). TG levels did not change in either sex. FFA concentration increased significantly in female rats from 10 days ($p < .001$). HDL-C concentration in female rats declined significantly from 10 days ($p < .01$) and remained low; in males it declined from 40 days ($p < .01$). LCAT activity showed a significant decrease from 10 days in females ($p < .001$), and from 20 days ($p < .001$) in males, remaining low until the end. The decrease in HDL-C and LCAT appeared to run in parallel in both sexes. The body weights did not change significantly. It is known that HDL-C plays a protective role against atherosclerosis and CHD. From our results, it appears that forced cold swimming up to 60 days results in significant decreases of HDL-C and LCAT, which may reflect adaptations of HDL-C metabolism. Cold stress, by lowering HDL-C and LCAT levels, may constitute a risk factor for CHD and atherosclerosis.

Effects of Exercise Intensity on Muscle Metabolism in Thyroidectomized Dogs

H. Kaciuba-Uściłko, B. Kruk, Z. Brzezińska, and K. Nazar

Department of Applied Physiology, Medical Research Centre, Polish Academy of Sciences, Warsaw, Poland

Body temperature (T_{re} and T_m)., oxygen uptake ($\dot{V}O_2$), heart rate (HR), and muscle metabolite content responses to 30-min bouts of treadmill exercise of different intensities (of approx. 40, 55, and 70 W) were compared in 7 dogs before (control-C) and then 6 weeks following surgical thyroidectomy (THY). At rest THY dogs had slightly lowered metabolic rate, HR, T_{re}, and T_m, whereas their muscle glycogen and lactate (LA) contents markedly exceeded the control levels. At each exercise intensity THY dogs reached lower $\dot{V}O_2$, HR, and body temperatures, but significant differences in comparison with C were found only at the highest work load (70 W). Muscle glycogen depletion was greater in THY than in C animals at the lowest exercise rate, but at the higher intensities it became considerably reduced. Muscle free glucose and hexose phosphate contents were lower, whereas muscle pyruvate (PA) and LA contents were elevated in THY dogs in comparison with controls at lower work loads but not at the highest intensity. At each of the exercise loads, muscle creatine phosphate (CrP) and ATP as well as the total adenine nucleotide decrements were more pronounced in THY than in C dogs.

In intact C dogs postexercise contents of muscle glycogen, CrP, and ATP were negatively correlated with work loads, while muscle PA, LA, and ADP concentrations showed a positive correlation. In THY dogs significant relationships with exercise intensity were found only for adenine nucleotides. Moreover, the correlation coefficients and the slopes of the regression lines, characterizing those relationships, were greater in comparison with those in C. This study suggests that in spite of high resting glycogen content in THY dogs there is a limitation of the substrate utilization during exercise, which results in an inability to provide fuel for ATP resynthesis at high exercise loads. This may be considered as one of the factors responsible for impairment of exercise tolerance in the thyroid hormone deficiency.

Part IV

Endocrine Responses to Exercise and Environmental Changes

Regional Cerebral Blood Flow, Neurotransmitters, and Cardiac Hormonal Reactions During Exercise

W. Hollmann, K. de Meirleir, K. Herholz, W.D. Heiss,
H. Bittner, K. Völker, and W.G. Forssmann
Institute for Cardiology and Sports Medicine, German Sports University,
Köln, F.R.G.

Current knowledge on the influence of exercise and training on the hemodynamics and metabolic processes of the human brain is rather limited. Modern techniques allow the first pertinent examinations. This paper deals with the two main points:

1. The cerebral blood flow during ergometer exercise of different intensities; and
2. The behavior of some neurotransmitters and of cardiodilatine during dosed exercise.

Cerebral Blood Flow During Ergometer Exercise

According to the general scientific opinion, the autonomous hemodynamic regulation of the brain guarantees a constant cerebral blood flow at least during light and moderate physical exercise (Heistad & Kontos, 1983; Herholz et al., 1987). On the other hand, some authors have described a local increase of blood flow in the pertinent brain sections when moving small muscle groups (Foreman et al., 1976; Globus et al., 1983; Gross et al., 1980; Ingvar & Philipson, 1977; Kleinerman & Sancetta, 1955; Lambertsen et al., 1959; Olesen, 1971; Pannier & Leusen, 1977; Roland et al., 1980; Zobl et al., 1965). This is the reason why we investigated the influence of different work loads during the ergometer exercise on regional cerebral blood flow in the left hemisphere.

Twelve healthy male human subjects between the ages of 20 and 30 years, with a mean maximum oxygen uptake of 3600 ± 250 ml • min^{-1}, were split into two groups. Six of them performed a bicycle exercise in a supine position at 25 W, the others at 100 W, over a period of 15 min. We used a modified ^{133}Xe method by injecting a bolus into the left cubital vein to measure the regional blood flow of the left hemisphere. The activity of the left hemisphere was monitored using a gamma camera system with a specially developed colliator combined with a computer (see Herholz et al., 1987).

Both the 25 W and 100 W loads resulted in a highly significant increase of cerebral blood flow in comparison with the initial values at rest. The method used allowed us to differentiate between the blood flow of the grey and the white brain matter. The total blood flow of the left hemisphere increased by 13.5% at 25 W and by 24.7% at 100 W. An increase of blood flow in the grey matter was 16.3% at 25 W and 27.3% at 100 W. At both work loads the blood flow increased significantly in all sections of the left hemisphere (the frontal, precentral, postcentral, parietal, temporal, and occipital lobe). In all these sections the blood flow increased much more in the grey than in the white matter (Figure 1).

"Cerebral autoregulation" means that an increase of the arterial blood pressure is compensated for by an augmentation of the cerebral vascular resistance. Thus, the cerebral blood flow can be maintained constant at the broad range of arterial blood pressure (between

CBF increase (%)

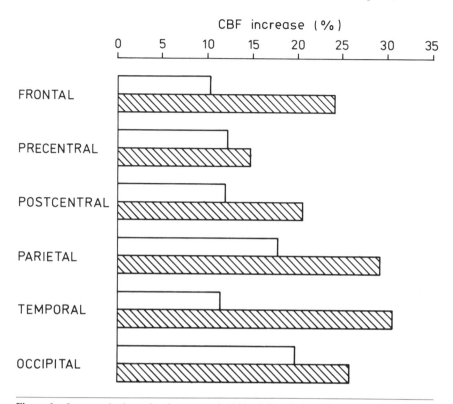

Figure 1. Increases in the regional mean cerebral blood flow during 25 (open bars) and 100 W (hatched bars) physical exercise in percentage of preexercise values (Herholz et al., 1987).

60 and 150 mmHg). Lately, however, it was found that an increase of the arterial blood pressure by 10 mmHg, under otherwise constant conditions, might cause an augmentation of the cerebral blood flow by about 6% in humans (Heistad & Kontos, 1983). The increases in the blood flow rate which we observed were only slightly greater than those that could be calculated from the above mentioned data. Moreover, the increased neuronal activity probably triggers an additional increase of the blood flow rate. Thus, an expansion of the local blood flow in the pertinent neuronal centers between 8% and 22.8% could be observed during the exercise performed by small muscle groups (Ingvar & Philipson, 1977; Oleson, 1971; Roland et al., 1980). On the other hand, measurements on miniature pigs (Foreman et al., 1984) or dogs (Gross et al., 1980; Pannier et al., 1977) exercising on a treadmill showed a constant or even slightly decreasing cerebral blood flow.

Probably the most important factor influencing the blood flow rate is pCO_2. It remains constant with light and moderate physical exercise and even decreases at the limits of maximal performance capacity (Hollmann, 1983; Hollmann & Hettinger, 1980). Thus, an increase in pCO_2 cannot be responsible for the increase of blood flow. The arterial pO_2 remains mostly unchanged or even increases slightly during work loads chosen in the present study; thus it cannot induce an augmentation in blood flow. We observed no preference of the blood flow increase in the pre- or postcentral section. This finding might admittedly be connected with the grouping structure of our regional detectors. The primary motor area for the legs is located near the interhemispheric fissure and accordingly it is rather remote from the surface gamma camera. Registration of smaller regions may possibly have allowed us to discover regional differences.

The findings collected so far led to the question whether other factors still unconsidered may be responsible for the increased cerebral blood flow during exercise. In the investigations described below we detected a considerable influence of brain neurohormones on the peripheral blood flow and the peripheral metabolism during physical exercise. Speculatively, one could therefore ask whether the increase of cerebral blood flow occurring even during light exercise may have the function of facilitating the transport of the hormones produced in the brain to the target organs in the body periphery.

Behavior of Some Neurotransmitters and of Cardiodilatine During Ergometer Exercise

The endogenous opioids first described in 1975 are traceable in the brain and in the peripheral blood. By using a specific radioimmunoassay (RIA) we found the plasma concentrations of β-endorphins between 10 and 20 ng • L^{-1} at rest (Arentz et al., 1986). Psychological and physical stress cause an increase in the blood endorphin level. We examined the significance of hemodynamic and metabolic aspects of physical work for the sensitivity and tolerance of pain as well as for the emotional condition. For this purpose studies were carried out with 10 healthy male subjects between 20 and 30 years of age. Each of them underwent three ergometer tests, with the work loads identical, on three different days. The first test served as a control. On the second and third day of examination either placebo (5 ml physiological saline solution) or 2 mg naloxone were injected into the cubital vein 5 min before the test. The succession of the placebo or naloxone tests was randomized, and they were carried out as a double blind test.

The work load was applied according to the Hollmann-Venrath standard testing method. After having started with 30 W, the intensity was increased every 3 min by 40 W up to the individual limits of performance capacity. Besides the usual spiroergometric data, we determined the arterial lactate level as well as the venous prolactin and ACTH levels. Additionally, the sublingual body temperature was checked.

To cause pain, we used a bipolar electric stimulus to the pulp of a healthy upper jaw incisor tooth without dental filling. An electrode-holding device made of synthetic material was produced to guarantee maximal reproductibility. For keeping the constant transitional resistance, we coated the stimulating electrodes with a conductive rubber material. For the electric impulses we used stimulation currents of 0.8 ms duration in intervals of one s each. The test persons' statements about their pain perception allowed us to assess the pain sensitivity threshold and pain tolerance threshold. The test persons had been familiarized with the following pain scaling a few days before the actual experiments: 0 = no perception, 1 = perception threshold, 2 = distinct perception, 3 = unpleasant perception, 4 = pain threshold, 5 = weak pain, 6 = distinct pain, 7 = strong pain, and 8 = intolerable pain. We used an individual condition scale ("Eigenzustandsskala") as a procedure to judge gradually the state of emotion and pain sensitivity.

No influence of endogenous opioids on oxygen uptake, respiratory minute volume, respiratory equivalent, heart rate, and systolic blood pressure could be traced. An unchanged sublingual temperature was noted in spite of the physical work. The blockade of the endogenous opioids by naloxone caused a highly significant decrease in the threshold of pain sensitivity and tolerance. Two mg naloxone were sufficient not only to neutralize the highly significant raise of the pain threshold and the tolerance threshold found under normal conditions after the maximal work load but even to shift them into the opposite direction. Moreover, wearing the respiratory mask and blood sampling from the earlobe were perceived as extremely unpleasant or even painful under the influence of naloxone (Figures 2 and 3).

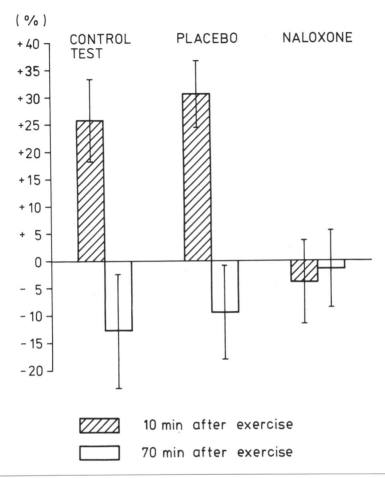

Figure 2. Changes in pain sensitivity 10 and 70 min after maximal physical exercise without any drug (control test), with placebo, and with naloxone. The values are related to basal conditions (Arentz et al., 1986).

The emotional condition after physical load improved distinctly under normal conditions, but deteriorated intensely under the influence of naloxone. According to de Meirleir et al. (1985) an exercise of intensity below the 4 mmol • L^{-1} lactate threshold does not trigger an increase of β-endorphins. The level of endogenous opioids increases highly significantly only after exceeding the aerobic-anaerobic threshold. Thus, the discrepancies in the literature concerning presence or absence of a "high" feeling after jogging might be explained by different intensities of jogging or other endurance exercises. The longing of endurance-trained athletes for ever more extreme workloads could be explained by the spill of endorphins hereby triggered. In extreme cases, a dependency on body-inherent morphines can be connected with the incidence of withdrawal symptoms like fear, depression, and irritability, as we were able to observe in one person.

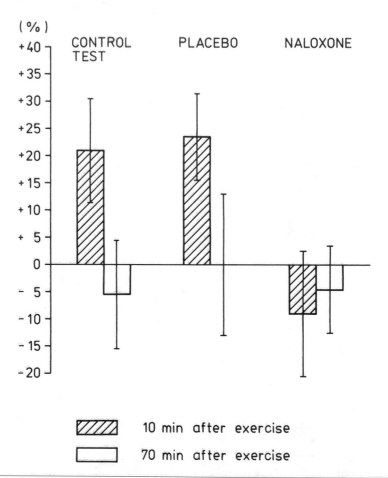

(%)

| | CONTROL TEST | PLACEBO | NALOXONE |

10 min after exercise

70 min after exercise

Figure 3. Changes in pain tolerance 10 and 70 min after maximal physical exercise without any drug (control test), with placebo, and with naloxone. The values are related to basal conditions (Arentz et al., 1986).

In further tests, de Meirleir et al. (1985) investigated the influence of serotonin and dopamine on hemodynamic and metabolic parameters during graded exercise. The serotonin tests were carried out with a blockade of the serotonin effect by ketanserine while the dopamine test with the dopamine agonist pergolide. The serotonin blockade did not change heart rate at rest or during exercise, but it did lower the arterial blood pressure during exercise. The maximum oxygen uptake remained unchanged. At the same time, the increase in the lactic acid level curve shifted to the right towards higher load intensities. ACTH and prolactin secretion induced by exercise was suppressed highly significantly (Figures 4 and 5).

Under the influence of the dopamine agonist pergolide, reduction of the systolic blood pressure and a decrease in norepinephrine and lactic acid levels at a given work load were found to be accompanied by lower heart rate. Generally, the dopamine agonist caused changes similar to the effect of endurance training. Simultaneously, the exercise-induced

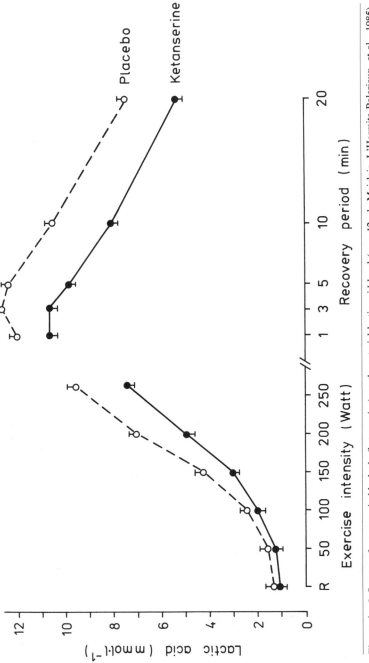

Figure 4. Influence of a serotonin blockade (ketanserine) on the arterial lactic acid level ($n = 12$; de Meirleir, L'Hermite-Baleriaux, et al., 1985).

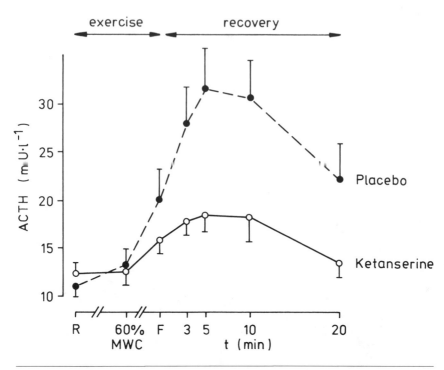

Figure 5. Changes in blood ACTH level during submaximal (60% MWC) and maximal (F) exercise under serotonin blockade with ketanserine (n = 12; de Meirleir, L'Hermite-Baleriaux, et al., 1985).

increases in blood prolactin and ACTH concentrations were suppressed. The causes of these changes are still unknown (Figures 6 and 7).

Cardiodilatine 126, a heart-muscle-produced hormone with a vascular dilatating effect, which was first described in detail in 1984 by Forssmann, is viewed today as being more and more connected with neurotransmitters. The hypothalamic region seems to exert a regulatory function even here. The cardiodilatine level in the blood increases with work load. The significance of this natriuretic hormone for the control of blood pressure during exercise is still unsettled.

In conclusion, dynamic work of large muscle groups causes a significant increase of cerebral blood flow even during light or moderate work intensities. This may enable a fast transport of neurotransmitters. The neurohormones affect regulatory processes in peripheral hemodynamics and in muscle metabolism. The detailed mechanisms are still largely unknown.

Acknowledgments

Supported by Bundesinstitut für Sportwissenschaft, Köln, by Wilder-Stiftung, and by the Prime Minister of NRW.

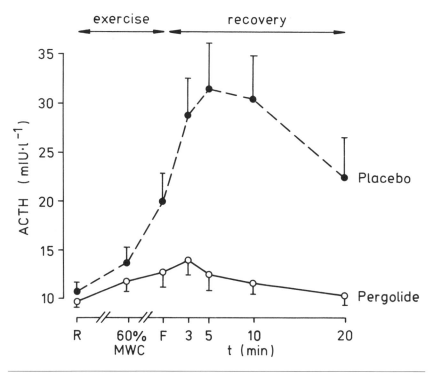

Figure 6. Influence of the dopamine agonist pergolide on blood ACTH level during sub-maximal (60% MWC) and maximal (F) physical exercise ($n = 12$; de Meirleir, Baeyens, L'Hermite, L'Hermite-Bateriaux, Olbrecht, & Hollmann 1985).

References

Arentz, T., de Meirleir, K., & Hollmann, W. (1986). Die Rolle der endogenen opioiden Peptide während Fahrradergometerarbeit. *Dtsch. Z. Sportmed.*, **37**, 210.

Bittner, H., Rippegather, G., Völker, K., Hollmann, W., & Forssmann, W.G. (1986). Freisetzung kardialer Hormone unter ergometrischer Belastung. *Dtsch. Z. Sportmed.*, **37**, 356.

de Meirleir, K., Arentz, T., Hollmann, W., & Vanhaelst, L. (1985). The role of endogenous opiates in thermal regulation of the body during exercise. *Brit. Med. J.*, **290**, 739.

de Meirleir, K., Baeyens, L., L'Hermite, M., L'Hermite-Baleriaux, M., & Hollmann, W. (1985). Exercise-induced prolactine release is related to anaerobiosis. *J. Clin. Endocrinol. Metab.*, **60**, 1.

de Meirleir, K., Baeyens, L., L'Hermite, M., L'Hermite-Baleriaux, M., Olbrecht, J., & Hollmann, W. (1985). *Pergolide mesylate inhibits exercise-induced prolactine release in man.* Internat. Congress Biochemistry, Copenhagen.

de Meirleir, K., L'Hermite-Baleriaux, M., L'Hermite, M., Rost, R., & Hollmann, W. (1985). Evidence for serotoninergic control of exercise-induced prolactine secretion. *Horm. Metab. Res.*, **17**, 379.

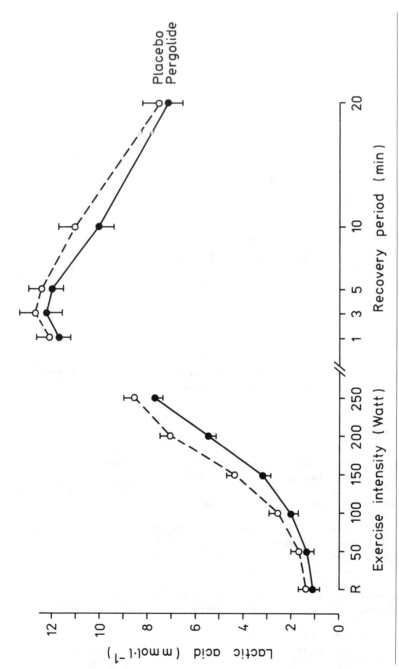

Figure 7. Effect of dopamine agonist pergolide on changes in the arterial lactic acid level during submaximal and maximal work loads ($n = 12$; de Meirleir, Baeyens, L'Hermite, L'Hermite-Bateriaux, Olbrecht, & Hollmann 1985).

Foreman, D.L., Sanders, M., & Bloor, C.M. (1976). Total and regional cerebral blood flow during moderate and severe exercise in miniature swine. *J. Appl. Physiol.*, **40**, 191.

Forssmann, W.G., Hock, D., Kirchheim, S., Metz, J., Mutt, V., & Reinicke, M. (1984). Cardiac hormones: Morphological and functional aspects. *Clin. and Expert. Theory and Practice*, **6**, 1873.

Globus, M., Melamed, E., Keren, A., Tzivoni, D., Granot, C., Lavy, S., & Stern, S. (1983). Effect of exercise on cerebral circulation. *J. Cereb. Blood Flow Metab.*, **3**, 287.

Gross, P.M., Marcus, M.L., & Heistad, D.D. (1980). Regional distribution of cerebral blood-flow during exercise in dogs. *J. Appl. Physiol.*, **48**, 213.

Heistad, D.D., & Kontos, H.A. (1983). Cerebral circulation. In *Handbook of Physiology*, (Sect. 2, Vol. III). American Physiol. Soc., Bethesda, Maryland, 137-182.

Herholz, K., Buskies, W., Rist, M., Pawlik, G., Hollmann, W., & Heiss, W.D. (1987). Regional cerebral blood flow in man at rest and during exercise. *J. Neurol.*, **234**, 9.

Hollmann, W. (1983). Körperliches Training und Hirnleistungs-insuffizienz-Terra incognita. *Therapiewoche*, **33**, 1584.

Hollmann, W., & Hettinger, Th. (1980). *Sportmedizin-Arbeits- und Trainingsgrundlagen.* Schattauer, Stuttgart-New York.

Ingvar, D.H., & Philipson, L. (1977). Distribution of cerebral blood flow in the dominant hemisphere during motor ideation and motor performance. *Ann. Neurol.*, **2**, 230.

Kleinerman, J., & Sancetta, S. (1955). Effect of mild steady state exercise on cerebral and general hemodynamics of normal untrained subjects. *J. Clin. Invest.*, **34**, 945.

Lambertsen, C.J., Owen, S.G., Vendel, H., Strood, M.W., Lurie, A.A., Lochner, W., & Clark, G.F. (1959). Respiratory and cerebral circulatory control during exercise at .21 and 2.0 atmospheres inspired pO_2. *J. Appl. Physiol.*, **14**, 966.

Olesen, J. (1971). Contralateral focal increase of cerebral blood-flow in man during arm work. *Brain*, **94**, 635.

Pannier, J.L., & Leusen, I. (1977). Regional blood flow in response to exercise in conscious dogs. *J. Appl. Physiol.*, **36**, 255.

Roland, P.E., Skinhoj, E., Lassen, N.A., & Larsen, B. (1980). Different cortical areas in man in organization of voluntary movements in extrapersonal space. *J. Neurophysiol.*, **43**, 137.

Zobl, E.G., Talmers, F.N., Christensen, R.C., & Baer, L.J. (1965). Effect of exercise on the cerebral circulation and metabolism. *J. Appl. Physiol.*, **20**, 1289.

Activity of the Pituitary–Adrenocortical System During Various Exercises

A. Viru, K. Karelson, T. Smirnova, and K. Port

Department of Sports Physiology and Laboratory of Hormonal Regulation of Muscular Activity, Tartu State University Tartu, U.S.S.R.

A great number of papers have been published on changes in the adrenocortical activity during various exercises. In most cases the results are rather variable and it is quite difficult to reveal the common responses (Galbo, 1983; Shephard & Sidney, 1975; Terjung, 1979; Tharp, 1975, Viru, 1985). In this paper, attention is going to be paid to the relationships between exercise intensity, its duration or the fitness of a person, and the dynamics of adrenocortical response.

Materials and Methods

The performed experiments and characteristics of subjects are summarized in Table 1. The venous blood samples were collected through a teflon catheter before, during, and after exercises performed under the laboratory conditions. Blood samples were also obtained before and after sports events, mentioned in Table 1. The plasma ACTH and cortisol (F) concentrations were determined by radioimmunoassays, using commercial kits. Blood lactate (LA) level was measured by the enzymatic method, and glucose using a Lachema (Czechoslovakia) kit.

Results and Discussion

During exercise of stepwise increasing intensity, an augmentation of the cortisol level in blood was found after the step that caused an increase in LA concentration over 4 mmol $\cdot$ L^{-1} (Table 2). Hence, the obtained results are in accordance with the opinion that the threshold for the activation of endocrine systems is within the same range of intensity as anaerobic threshold (Lehmann et al., 1981; Viru, 1985). Further increase in exercise intensity did not cause any significant increase in blood cortisol concentration. After the spurt, performed at the level of the highest possible power output, in many cases the cortisol concentration was below values obtained after graded exercise. The results agree with data of Barwich et al. (1982), suggesting that a high level of hydrogen ions may suppress cortisol secretion.

Untrained students were able to perform exercise at 85% of their $\dot{V}O_2$max during 779 $\pm$ 40 s and at 140% of $\dot{V}O_2$max for 99 $\pm$ 7 s. After the exercises, blood LA levels were 12.6 $\pm$ 0.7 and 7.3 $\pm$ 0.6 mmol $\cdot$ L^{-1}, respectively. Thus, the more prolonged exercise resulted in more pronounced anaerobic glycogenolysis despite the lower power output. Mild hyperglycemia was detected only after the more prolonged exercise. Only such an anaerobic exercise caused a significant activation of pituitary-adrenocortical system in all

Table 1   Performed Experiments and Characteristics of Subjects

Subjects	No. of persons	Age (years)	$\dot{V}O_2$max (ml • min⁻¹ • kg⁻¹)	Type of exercise
Moderately trained skiers	6	19-22	50.6 ± 1.4	Exercise of stepwise increased intensity on bicycle ergometer (after every 4 min the intensity increased by 50 W; the exercise was finished by a 1-min spurt at the highest possible power output)
Untrained students	13	22.6 ± 0.7	50.6 ± 1.5	Exercises on the bicycle ergometer at 85 and 140% of $\dot{V}O_2$max to exhaustion
Untrained students	9	21-25		A 30-min intensive strength exercise
Untrained students and endurance athletes	56	17-35	40-89	2-hour exercise on a bicycle ergometer at 44-76% of $\dot{V}O_2$max
Various subjects	42	18-33		Cross-country run for 20 km
Various subjects	18	14-51		60-km skiing marathon
Athletes	7	33 ± 3		Triathlon (38 km of swimming, 180 km of cycling, 42 km of running)
Athletes	14	29 ± 3		Short triathlon (1.5 km of swimming, 42 km of cycling, 14 km of running)
Trained runners	9	51.9 ± 1.3		1000-km run during 15 days

subjects (Table 3). Thus, during the over-threshold exercises the activation of this endocrine system is related to the rate of anaerobic glycogenolysis rather than to the actual intensity of exercise.

It may be assumed that exercises performed to increase strength should not activate the pituitary-adrenocortical system as they do not cause any marked increase in lactate accumulation. However, the applied program of intensive strength exercises was found to cause a significant elevation in the plasma corticotropin and cortisol levels (Table 4). Corticotropin concentration returned to the initial value within 1 h and cortisol concentration within 6 h. In the period of 6-24 h after cessation of exercises the corticotropin and cortisol levels were below the initial values. After strength exercises a mild hyperglycemia, persisting up to the 6th hour of the recovery period, was noted.

Table 2 Blood Cortisol and Lactate Levels During Exercise With Stepwise Increasing (After Every 4 Min) Intensity

Intensity of exercise	0	100 W	150 W	200 W	250 W	300 W	Spurt
Cortisol (nm • L^{-1})	440	493	417	477	540	648	495
	±38	±19	±33	±32	±39	±38	±50
Lactate (mm • L^{-1})	1.30	2.49	4.20	4.33	5.85	6.30	10.70
	∓0.11	∓0.08	±0.76	±0.31	±0.72	±0.47	±0.36

Note. M ± SE.

Table 3 Blood Corticotropinn and Cortisol Levels After the Exercise of Maximal Duration, Performed at 85 and 140% of $\dot{V}O_2$max

	Corticotropin (pg • ml^{-1})				Cortisol (nm • L^{-1})			
	Before	Just after	15 min after	30 min after	Before	Just after	15 min after	30 min after
85% of $\dot{V}O_2$max	46	132	67	53	410	480	713	700
	±15	±29	±17	±18	±37	±45	±37	±56
140% of $\dot{V}O_2$max	22	34	28	13	465	480	464	459
	± 6	±12	± 4	± 2	±43	±35	±58	±71

Note. M ± SE.

Table 4 Blood Corticotropin and Cortisol Levels After a 30-Min Intensive Strength Exercise

	Before	Just after	1 h after	6 h after	24 h after
Corticotropin (pg • ml^{-1})	21 ± 5	116 ± 17	22 ± 8	16 ± 3	12 ± 2
Cortisol (nm • L^{-1})	633 ± 40	900 ± 47	950 ± 65	437 ± 27	482 ± 52

Note. M ± SE.

During 2-hour exercise on a bicycle ergometer, four different variants of dynamics in blood in blood cortisol concentrations can be distinguished:

1. A preliminary increase followed by a decrease down to the initial level or below it (7 subjects), after 20 to 30 min of exercise;

2. a biphasic increase—peak values noted during the first 30 min and then at the end of exercise with a decrease after the first peak (26 subjects);
3. the lack of alterations or a moderate decrease during the first 20 to 60 min of exercise with a pronounced elevation during the second hour of exercise (14 subjects); and
4. a decrease during the whole period of exercise (9 subjects).

The persons revealing various variants of dynamics did not differ significantly among themselves in $\dot{V}O_2$max, the relative intensity of exercise (% of $\dot{V}O_2$max) or the initial level of blood cortisol. The initial concentration of blood glucose or its dynamics during exercise did not differ, and it was impossible to correlate any of the above mentioned differences with the effect of the glucostatic mechanism (Kozłowski & Nazar, 1979).

In 8 subjects the 2-hour exercise was repeated 2 to 3 times over a period of a year at the same level of intensity. In most cases the cortisol dynamics were identical. Only when the intensity of exercise was substantially decreased, then the biphasic increase changed into a decrease during the whole period of exercise. However, in other subjects who showed an overall decrease in blood cortisol levels, an increase in exercise intensity did not change the hormone dynamics. Thus, the occurrence of different variants of dynamics seems to depend on the stable individual properties of a person.

In most cases the alterations in corticotropin level were characterized by a biphasic increase (peak values during the first 20 min of exercise and at the end of exercise). Thus, the dynamics of corticotropin and cortisol levels coincided only in the second variant of the former. In the first variant the adrenal cortex responded to the first corticotropin peak and in the third variant only to the second one. In the fourth variant the corticotropin peaks did not coincide with the adrenocortical response.

These data indicate that prolonged exercise activated the pituitary-adrenocortical system, but in a number of cases a blockade of adrenocortical response to corticotropin was noted. This kind of blockade may occur at the level of corticotropin receptors on the membrane of adrenocorticocytes, at the level of postreceptor events of the corticotropin action, and at the level of the enzymes, catalyzing various steps of cortisol biosynthesis. There is no data that allows us to prefer any of these possibilities, or exclude any others. The meaning of the described blockade also remains unclear. However, it is reasonable to suggest that during prolonged exercise a pronounced variability in alterations of cortisol levels is caused by the lack of or occurrence of the blockade of adrenocortical response to corticotropin.

The bursts of corticotropin secretion at the beginning of exercise and also after some period of exercise suggest that the activation of the pituitary-adrenocortical system may be determined by two thresholds: exercise intensity (determining the activation at the beginning of exercise) and exercise duration (becoming decisive after a certain time of exercise). If the first activation is of a short duration, then the activation after exceeding the duration threshold becomes stable and prolonged. This has been expressed by the high level of blood cortisol obtained after various sports events of long duration (Dessypris et al., 1976; Keul et al, 1981; Maron et al., 1975). Accordingly, our results showed very high levels of cortisol in blood after 20 km of cross-country running, 60 km of skiing, and a competitive triathlon. However, during a run of 1000 km with daily distances of 60 to 100 km no elevation in the blood cortisol level was observed. It is necessary in this case to maintain a low intensity of exercise from the beginning to be able to perform successfully exercises of very long duration. The pituitary-adrenocortical system may not be activated under such conditions.

Conclusion

During exercise, activation of the pituitary-adrenocortical system depends on the intensity and duration thresholds (Figure 1). The first threshold is within the same range of intensity

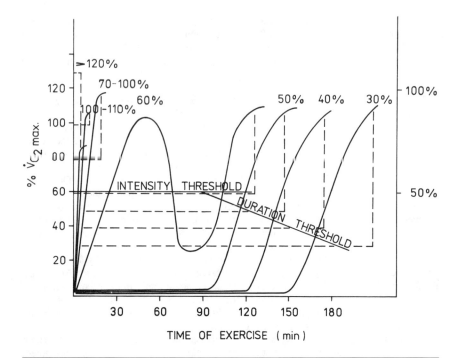

Figure 1. Intensity and duration thresholds for activation of the pituitary-adrenocortical system. Left ordinate as well as % values on the figure indicate % of VO₂max, whereas the right ordinate shows a degree of activation of pituitary-adrenocortical system.

as the anaerobic threshold. During exercise of intensity exceeding this threshold the activation of this endocrine system is related rather to the rate of anaerobic glycogenolysis than to exercise intensity by itself. However, during an intensive strength exercise, activation of the system occurs without any pronounced lactate accumulation. Thus, the intensity threshold differs in meaning in various types of exercise.

When long-term exercise is performed the duration threshold is achieved. Then the activity of the pituitary-adrenocortical system increases although the intensity did not reach the threshold level. Probably, the lower the exercise intensity, the longer must the exercise last to reach the duration threshold. However, there is a minimal level of intensity below which the duration threshold does not exist. When the exercise intensity is over the threshold value, the duration threshold results in the subsequent activation of the pituitary-adrenocortical system.

References

Barwich, D., Rettenmeier, A., & Weicker, A. (1982). Serum levels in the so called "stress hormones" in athletes after short consecutive exercise. *Int. J. Sports Med.* (Suppl. 22). World Congress of Sport Med., 8.

Dessypris, A., Kuoppasalmi, K., & Adlercreuz, H. (1976). Plasma cortisol, testosterone, androstenedione and luteinizing hormone (LH) in a non-competitive marathon run. *J. Steroid Biochem., 7*, 33-37.

Galbo, H. (1983). *Hormonal and metabolic adaptation to exercise.* G. Thieme, Verlag, Stuttgart.

Keul, J., Kohler, B., von Glutz, G., Luthi, U., & Howald, H. (1981). Biochemical changes in a 100-km run: Carbohydrates, lipids, and hormones in serum. *Eur. J. Appl. Physiol.,* **47**, 181-189.

Kozłowski, S., & Nazar, K. (1979). Physiological regulation of exercise metabolism. *Acta Physiol. Pol.,* **30**(Suppl. 18), 19-61.

Lehmann, M., Keul, J., Huber, G., & Da Orada, M. (1981). Plasma catecholamines in trained and untrained volunteers during graduated exercise. *Int. J. Sports Med.,* **2**, 143-147.

Maron, M.B., Horvath, S.M., & Wilkerson, J.E. (1975). Acute blood biochemical alterations in response to marathon running. *Eur. J. Appl. Physiol.,* **34**, 173-181.

Shephard, R.J., & Sidney, K.H. (1975). Effects of physical exercise on plasma growth hormone and cortisol levels in human subjects. *Exercise and Sport Sciences Reviews,* **3**, 1-30.

Terjung, R.L. (1979). Endocrine response to exercise. *Exercise and Sport Sciences Reviews,* **7**, 153-180.

Tharp, G.P. (1975). The role of glucocorticoids in exercise. *Med. Sci. Sports.,* **7**, 6-11.

Viru, A. (1985). *Hormones in muscular activity. Vol. I. Hormones in Exercise.* CRC Press, Boca Raton.

Role of the Thyroid Gland in Adaptation to the Environment

D.L. Ingram and M.J. Dauncey

Institute of Animal Physiology and Genetics Research, Babraham, Cambridge, U.K.

Adaptation to environmental temperature has for many years been associated with changes in thyroid metabolism. Among the earliest studies was that of Starr and Roskelly (1940), who showed that the height of the secretory thyroidal epithelium in rats exposed to cold was greater than that of those in the warm. The conclusion that environmental temperature affects the thyroid gland has also been recorded in other species (Eastman et al., 1974; Ingram & Slebodzinski, 1968). The immediate response to cold exposure is now also known to involve the secretion of TSH (Reichlin et al., 1972). Moreover, local cooling of the hypothalamus leads to increased secretion from the thyroid gland (Andersson et al., 1962).

In the young growing pig the secretion of thyroxine (T_4) in response to local cooling of the hypothalamus was demonstrated by Evans & Ingram (1974). The immediate effect of a reduction in ambient temperature from 32 to 8 °C was also shown to be a rise in the plasma concentration of T_4 (Evans & Ingram, 1977). However, the increased concentration persisted for only a few days in the cold when food intake was restricted to that taken at 32 °C. The fractional disappearance rate (k) at which radioactively labeled T_4 was lost from the blood when pigs were transferred from 32 to 8 °C and given extra food also increased; but when food intake was kept constant, k did not change. The influence of food intake on the k value of T_4 has also been demonstrated in pigs kept at thermal neutrality (Ingram & Kaciuba-Uścilko, 1977). Further studies (Ingram & Dauncey, 1980) have shown that the value of k depends not only on energy intake, but also on the nutrient composition of the food. The addition of bran, which increased faecal bulk without changing the metabolizable energy intake, did not however affect the value of k. This latter point suggests that the effect of an increase in food intake does not depend on loss of T_4 by the entero-hepatic circulation.

The more active form of thyroid hormone is 3,5,3'-triiodothyronine (T_3) which is secreted from the thyroid gland in pigs (Slebodzinski et al., 1985) as well as in other species, and is also formed from T_4 by peripheral 5' monodeiodination. The alternative product from T_4 is 3, 3', 5'-triiodothyronine (reverse T_3), which is biologically inactive. The rate of loss of T_4 thus does not necessarily run parallel to the metabolically active hormone. In the pig the value of k for T_3 was not changed by food intake, although that for reverse T_3 decreased on a low intake, suggesting that, as in man, there is a reduced deiodination of the 5' position during food deprivation which would affect T_4 and reverse T_3, but not T_3 (Ingram & Ramsden, 1981).

As a result of these studies, a re-examination of the long-term effects of cold on the thyroid gland had been made. It was found that in all earlier studies, although food composition had been kept constant, intake had been allowed to increase in the cold. Comparisons had therefore involved animals in the warm on a low food intake and those in the cold on a high food intake. The effects of ambient temperature and energy intake on young pigs were therefore studied in animals kept at 10 or 35 °C, and at both temperatures one group of pigs received twice as much food (H) as the other (L) producing four groups:

35H, 35L, 10H, and 10L (Dauncey & Ingram, 1986b; Ingram & Dauncey, 1986). The height of the epithelium of the thyroid gland was measured and found to be greater on an H intake than L, but there was no effect of temperature (Dauncey et al., 1984).

In further experiments, plasma concentrations of T_3 and T_4 were measured as well as their fractional disappearance rates, all blood samples being taken in a period several hours after feeding (Macari et al., 1983). The plasma concentrations of both T_3 and T_4 were greater on H than L intake, but again environmental temperature had no effect. By contrast the values of k for T_3 or T_4 were not affected by energy intake, but were greater at 10 than 35 °C. The catabolic rate of a hormone, that is, the quantity metabolized in unit time, depends on the product of the concentration, the k value, and the distribution volume. Consequently the catabolic rates were greater both on H than L (because of the difference in concentration); and at 10 than 35 °C (because of the difference in k). These findings on plasma concentration are in agreement with those from the histological study. The difference in k values however contrasts with the findings of Evans and Ingram (1977) and Ingram and Kaciuba-Uściłko (1977) in which it was found that energy intake did influence the k value for T_4. The effects of intake on the k values for T_3 and T_4 have therefore been examined in pigs during successive weeks after a change in energy intake at a constant ambient temperature (Griggio & Ingram, 1985). The results of this study confirmed that k for T_4 is initially increased when energy intake is increased, but that the effect is lost after about 4 weeks and the k value for T_3 is not significantly changed. It thus appears that the processes by which the thyroid gland adapts to changes in energy intake and environmental temperature are complex and alter with time.

The response of the thyroid hormone system to energy intake alone has also been examined by assay of plasma hormone concentrations of T_3 and T_4 before and after a single meal in young pigs fed once a day. In these studies (Dauncey et al., 1982; Dauncey et al., 1983) it was found that T_3 increased within an hour of eating a meal, and that the rise was greater after a large than a small intake. There was also a rise in T_4, although this was much slower and was not detected in pigs fed a low intake. Recent results (Dauncey & Ingram, unpublished) have shown that both total and free T_3 and T_4 are affected by eating a meal, but that a meal of large bulk, with negligible metabolizable energy content, is without effect.

Attention has also been paid to the effects of a single meal on the values of k. For T_3, which has a half-life of about 3 h in young pigs, the k value is significantly greater 1 to 3 h after than 22 to 24 h after, and since plasma concentration increases after a meal, the catabolic rate of T_3 is also increased by eating. The situation with respect to T_4 is more complex, since it was found that eating a meal caused a redistribution of the T_4 pool within the body and a change in the apparent distribution volume, which made it impossible to obtain a meaningful estimate of k in the period immediately after eating (Dauncey & Ingram, 1986a). These results drew attention to the importance of the times at which blood samples are taken for the determination of k value and plasma hormone concentration. In earlier studies (Evans & Ingram, 1977; Ingram & Kaciuba-Uściłko, 1977) samples for k values were taken over a 14 h period, and some errors due to the redistribution of the hormone pool during feeding would most likely have been encountered.

The response of an animal to T_3 depends not only on the concentration of hormone present, but also on the number of hormone receptors. Nuclear T_3 receptor numbers in the skeletal muscle of pigs from groups 35H, 35L, 10H, and 10L have therefore been measured (Dauncey et al., 1988). It was found that the greatest number of receptors occurred in the 35H group and the least in 10L with the 35L and 10H groups being intermediate and similar to each other. Consequently, both a cold environment and a low energy intake had significant effects in depressing receptor numbers. These findings imply that, contrary to expectation, a cold environment would reduce tissue responsiveness to thyroid hormones. It is known that starvation in rats leads to a reduction in receptor numbers (Samuels et al., 1983), and it seems probable that a low energy intake in relation to energy requirement may have been an important factor in this study on pigs. Thus, cold increases the use of energy and the same absolute quantity of energy intake would be smaller in relation to demand in animals at 10 °C than for those at 35 °C. Hence the 10L animals were relatively underfed by comparison with the 35L, and the 35H were relatively overfed by comparison with the 10H. The responsiveness of tissues to T_3 now needs to be tested in animals kept under different conditions of environment and energy intake. The conclusion which must be drawn from these studies is that although a cold environment has an immediate effect on stimulating the thyroid gland, in the long term both the metabolism of thyroid hormones and the number of hormone receptors are influenced to a large extent by the energy intake that is available.

References

Andersson, B., Ekman, L., Gale, C.C., & Sundsten, J.W. (1962). Thyroidal response to local cooling of the 'heat-loss centre'. *Acta Physiologica Scandinavica*, 63, 186-192.

Dauncey, M.J., Ingram, D.L., Macari, M., & Ramsden, D.B. (1982). Increase in plasma concentrations of thyroid hormones in piglets after a meal. *Journal of Physiology, London*, 327, 90-91P.

Dauncey, M.J., Ramsden, D.B., Kapadi, A.L., Macari, M., & Ingram, D.L. (1983). Increase in plasma concentrations of 3,5,3'-triiodothyronine and thyroxine after a meal, and its dependence on energy intake. *Hormone and Metabolic Research*, 15, 499-502.

Dauncey, M.J., Ingram, D.L., & Macari, M. (1984). Histology of the thyroid gland in animals living under different conditions of energy intake and environmental temperature. *Journal of Thermal Biology*, 9, 153-157.

Dauncey, M.J., & Ingram, D.L. (1986a). Influence of a single meal on fractional disappearance and catabolic rates of 3,5,3'-triiodothyronine and thyroxine over 24 hours. *Comparative Biochemistry & Physiology*, 83A, 89-92.

Dauncey, M.J., & Ingram, D.L. (1986b). Acclimatization to warm or cold temperatures and the role of food intake. *Journal of Thermal Biology*, 11, 89-93.

Dauncey, M.J., Brown, D., Hayashi, M., & Ingram, D.L. (1988). Thyroid hormone nuclear receptors in skeletal muscle as influenced by environmental temperature and energy intake. *Quarterly Journal of Experimental Physiology*, 73, 183-191.

Eastman, C.J., Eakins, R.P., Leith, I.M., & Williams, E.S. (1974). The thyroid response to prolonged cold exposure in man. *Journal of Physiology, London*, 241, 175-181.

Evans, S.E., & Ingram, D.L. (1974). The significance of deep body temperature in regulating the concentration of thyroxine in the plasma of the pig. *Journal of Physiology, London*, 236, 159-170.

Evans, S.E., & Ingram, D.L. (1977). The effect of ambient temperature upon the secretion of thyroxine in the young pig. *Journal of Physiology, London*, 264, 511-521.

Griggio, M.A., & Ingram, D.L. (1985). Effect of long term differences in energy intake on metabolic rate and thyroid hormones. *Hormone and Metabolic Research*, 17, 67-71.

Ingram, D.L., & Slebodzinski, A. (1968). Oxygen consumption and thyroid gland activity during adaptation to high ambient temperature in young pigs. *Research in Veterinary Science*, 6, 522-530.

Ingram, D.L., & Kaciuba-Uścitko, H. (1977). The influence of food intake and ambient temperature on the rate of thyroxine utilization. *Journal of Physiology, London*, 270, 431-438.

Ingram, D.L., & Dauncey, M.J. (1980). Effects of dietary composition on energy metabolism and rate of utilization of thyroxine. In L.E. Mount (Ed.), *Energy metabolism*. Butterworths, London, 411-415.

Ingram, D.L., & Ramsden, D.B. (1981). The influence of energy intake on metabolism of 3,5,3' triiodothyronine and 3,3',5' triiodothyronine in young pigs. *Journal of Endocrinology*, 88, 141-146.

Ingram, D.L., & Dauncey, M.J. (1986). Environmental effects on growth and development. In P.J. Buttery, N.B. Haynes, & D.B. Lindsay (Eds.), *Control and manipulation of animal growth*. Butterworths, London, 5-20.

Macari, M., Dauncey, M.J., Ramsden, D.B., & Ingram, D.L. (1983). Thyroid hormone metabolism after acclimatization to a warm or cold temperature under conditions of high or low energy intake. *Quarterly Journal of Experimental Physiology, 68*, 709-718.

Reichlin, S., Martin, J.B., Mitnich, M.A., Boshans, R.L., Grimm, Y., Bollinger, J., Gordon, J., & Malacara, J. (1972). The hypothalamus in pituitary thyroid regulation. *Recent Progress in Hormone Research, 28*, 229-286.

Samuels, H.H., Perlman, A.J., Raaka, B.M., & Stanley, F. (1983). Thyroid hormone receptor synthesis and degradation and interaction with chromatin components. In J.H. Oppenheimer & H.H. Samuels (Eds.), *Molecular basis of thyroid hormone action*. Academic Press, New York & London.

Slebodzinski, A.B., Ingram, D.L., & Dauncey, M.J. (1985). Conversion of thyroxine into 3,5,3'-triiodothyronine and 3,3',5'-triiodothyronine in the young pig. *Comparative Biochemistry and Physiology, 80A*, 559-563.

Starr, P., & Roskelly, R. (1940). A comparison of the effects of thyrotropic hormone on the thyroid gland. *American Journal of Physiology, 130*, 549-556.

RESEARCH NOTES

Hormonal Responses to Physical and Psychological Stressors in Exercising Rats

A. Dubaniewicz, D. Ježowa, and M. Vigaš

Department of Applied Physiology, Medical Research Centre, Polish Academy of Sciences, Warsaw, Poland and Institute of Experimental Endocrinology, Slovak Academy of Sciences, Bratislava, Czechoslovakia

It is not clear to what extent hormonal changes accompanying physical activity in animals are related to exercise per se, and to what extent to the stressful elements of experimental procedure caused by handling, noise, and so on. Recently, much attention has been paid to the effects of various stressors on the endocrine system (Eger et al., 1986; Kvetňanský et al., 1985; Sadjak et al., 1983; Vigaš, 1985). The above studies concerned mainly secretion of hormones being considered the typical "stress hormones" (Axelrod & Reisine, 1984), such as catecholamines, ACTH, and corticosteroids, while relatively less is known about effects of stressful events on insulin (IRI), thyroxine (T_4), and triiodothyronine (T_3) secretion. Thus, the aim of the present study was to distinguish the effects of acute exercise or physical training on the plasma concentrations of ACTH, IRI, T_4, and T_3 from the changes occurring in resting animals subjected to some emotional stimuli associated with exercise experiments.

Materials and Methods

The experiments were performed on 46 male Wistar rats divided into three groups: (1) control animals (C) kept in an animal house, five per cage, for the whole period of experiment (4 weeks) and then sacrificed there by decapitation ($n = 6$); (2) trained animals (T) carried to the laboratory five times a week and submitted to the training program consisting of 60-min treadmill running with speed 20 m • min^{-1} (slope 0°) for 4 weeks ($n = 20$); (3) rats exposed to some stress stimuli (S) connected with training (i.e., transferred to the laboratory together with T rats and exposed to noise of the treadmill, handling, etc.) ($n = 20$). At the end of the training program both T and S groups were divided into the following subgroups: (T_0) sacrificed 24 h after the last exercise bout; (T_E30) sacrificed after 30 min exercise; (T_E60) sacrificed after 60 min exercise; (S_1) sacrificed in the animal house; (S_2) sacrificed in the laboratory; ($S_{2E}30$) sacrificed in the laboratory after 30 min exercise of the same intensity as that performed by T_E30 rats. Immediately after decapitation blood was taken for radioimmunoassay determinations of ACTH, insulin (IRI), thyroxine (T_4), and triiodothyronine (T_3). Glucose and total cholesterol were measured enzymatically.

Results

At the end of the experiment body mass of trained rats was lower than that of the remaining groups. Plasma ACTH concentration did not differ significantly between groups at rest. The levels of this hormone determined in blood taken from rats exercising 30 min were, however, significantly lower in T than in S_2e group (Figure 1). Plasma insulin concentration in T rats at rest was significantly lower from the values in the remaining groups but there were no differences between the groups in the postexercise IRI. Only in untrained rats (S_2) exercise caused a significant decrease in the hormone concentration (Figure 2). Neither at rest nor after exercise did BG values differ between groups. Plasma thyroxine concentration (T_4) was significantly diminished in T rats at rest in comparison with C and S groups, while the level of T_4 in S rats was elevated above the control value. Exercise caused an increase in T_4 concentration only in trained rats (Figure 3). Plasma triiodothyronine (T_3) concentration at rest was significantly reduced in trained rats. Exercise did not influence the hormone level in either group (Figure 4). Plasma total cholesterol at rest was slightly but significantly elevated in T and S groups in comparison with control values. Exercise reduced plasma cholesterol level in T and S groups.

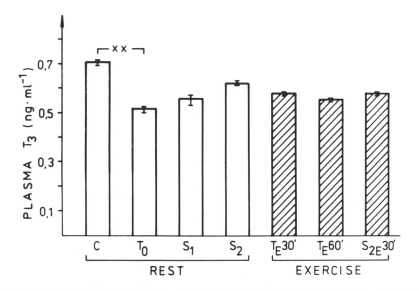

Figure 1. Comparison of ACTH concentration in trained rats and in rats exposed to stress stimuli (S) at rest and after physical exercise. *$p < .05$. T_O-sacrificed 24 h after the last exercise bout, S_1-sacrificed in the animal house, S_2-sacrificed in the laboratory, T_E30-sacrificed after 30 min exercise, T_E60-sacrificed after 60 min exercise, S_{2E}30-sacrificed in the laboratory after 30 min exercise of the same intensity as that performed by T_E30 rats.

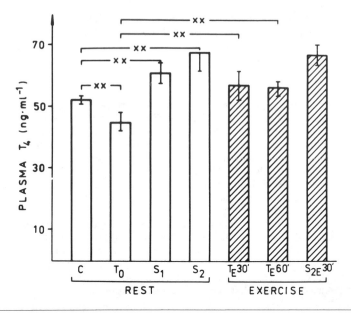

Figure 2. Comparison of insulin (IRI) concentration in control (C), trained (T), and exposed to stress stimuli (S) rats at rest and after physical exercise. Denotations as in Figure 2.

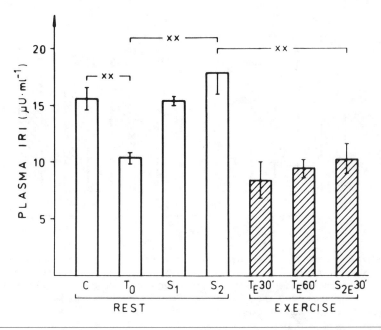

Figure 3. Comparison of thyroxine (T_4) concentration in control (C), trained (T), and exposed to stress stimuli (S) rats at rest and after physical exercise. Denotations as in Figure 2.

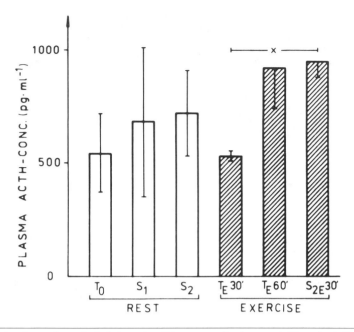

Figure 4.   Comparison of triiodothyronine (T₃) concentration in control (C), trained (T), and exposed to stress stimuli (S) rats at rest and after physical exercise. Denotations as in Figure 2.

Conclusion

These data indicate that the decreases in circulating insulin and thyroid hormone (T₃ and T₄) concentrations occurring in trained animals can be considered as specific effects of physical activity. Training does not affect specifically basal ACTH secretion but seems to cause an attenuation of the hormone response to exercise.

Acknowledgments

This work was partly supported by the Polish Central Programme for Basic Research 06-02.

References

Axelrod, J., & Reisine, D. (1984). Stress hormones: Their interaction and regulation. *Science, 224*, 452-459.

Eger, G., Sadjak, A., Porta, S., Supanz, S., & Pürstner, P. (1986). Laboratory handling and its influence on hormonal and metabolic parameters during acute inflammation in rats: A critique of long-term treatment by repeated injections *Horm. Metabol. Res., 18*, 746-749.

Kvetňanskỳ, R., Nemeth, Š., Vigaš, M., Opršalovà, Z., & Jurčovičovà, J. (1985). Plasma catecholamines in rats during adaptation to intermittent exposure to different stressors (1984). In E. Usdin, R. Kvetňanskỳ, & J. Axelrod (Eds.), *Stress*. Gordon & Breach Science Publishers, New York, 109-123.

Sadjak, A., Klingenberg, H.G., Egger, G., & Supanz, S. (1983). Evaluation of the effects of blood smelling, handling, and anesthesia on plasma catecholamines in rats. *Z. Versuchstierk, 25,* 245-250.

Vigaš, M. (1985). *Neuroendokrinńá reakcia v strese u človeka.* Veda, Bratislava.

Regulation of Hormonal Changes and Glucose Turnover in Humans During Exercise: Evidence for the Role of Motor Center Activity

M. Kjaer, N.H. Secher, and H. Galbo
Department of Medical Physiology B, Panum Institute and Department of Anaesthesia and Medicine, Rigshospitalet, University of Copenhagen, Denmark

Influence of feedback mechanisms on the hormonal response to exercise has been amply demonstrated (Galbo, 1983). However, during exercise mobilization of substrate energy stores may exceed needs suggesting that the endocrine system and substrate mobilization may be influenced by direct stimulation from motor centers (central command). The study evaluated the role of motor center activity for hormonal changes and substrate mobilization in exercising man. A small dose of d-tubocurarine was used to induce a partial neuromuscular blockade which, compared to control experiments, reduces muscle strength and necessitates a higher activity in motor centers during a given work load.

Methods

Eight young, healthy males (25 (23-37) years, 72 (62-80) kg, and 180 (170-186) cm (mean and range)) bicycled for two 20-min periods without (C) as well as during partial neuromuscular blockade with tubocurarine (Cu). C and Cu experiments were separated by 5 to 15 days. Arterialized blood was sampled from a heated hand vein; glucose turnover was measured by 3-^{3}H-glucose infusion and plasma catecholamine concentration determined by a single isotope radioenzymatic method. During exercise the intensity of effort was evaluated by rating of perceived exertion on a scale from 0 to 20 (arbitrary units).

Results

In the first exercise period $\dot{V}O_2$ (56% $\dot{V}O_2$max) and blood lactate (Table 1) were identical in Cu compared to C experiments, whereas hand grip strength was lower (reduced to approx. 66% of control) and rating of perceived exertion higher in Cu experiments (14 (12-17) vs 9 (6-12) points in C (median and range), $p < 0.01$), indicating higher motor center activity. Concentrations of norepinephrine, epinephrine, GH, and ACTH attained higher values in Cu than in C experiments (Table 1). The initial increase in glucose production (R_a) was enhanced in Cu compared to C, and plasma glucose increased only in Cu experiments ($p < .05$). FFA and glycerol concentrations were higher in Cu than in C experiments (Table 1). In the second exercise period identical perceived exertion was achieved in the two experiments by reducing work load in Cu experiments. In this period hormonal responses were similar in the two experiments (data not shown).

Table 1   Hormones and Metabolites at the End of 20 Min Exercise

	Tubocurarine (Cu)	Control (C)
$\dot{V}O_2$ (L $\cdot$ min^{-1})	2.22 $\pm$ 0.12	2.13 $\pm$ 0.12
Growth hormone (mU $\cdot$ L^{-1})	25.9 $\pm$ 7.3*	11.5 $\pm$ 4.7
ACTH (pmol $\cdot$ L^{-1})	11.3 $\pm$ 1.3*	5.5 $\pm$ 0.7
FFA (mmol $\cdot$ L^{-1})	0.64 $\pm$ 0.10*	0.53 $\pm$ 0.07
Glycerol (mmol $\cdot$ L^{-1})	0.18 $\pm$ 0.02**	0.15 $\pm$ 0.02
Lactate (mmol $\cdot$ L^{-1})	2.85 $\pm$ 0.75	2.84 $\pm$ 0.50

Note. Plasma concentrations obtained in response to bicycling at 56% $\dot{V}O_2$max (period 1) with (Cu) as well as without (C) partial neuromuscular blockade in 8 subjects. Values are mean $\pm$ *SE.* * and ** denote differences ($p < .05$ and $p < .1$, respectively) between curare and control experiments.

Discussion

Higher motor center activity in the first work period during curarization compared to control experiments was accompanied by higher response of catecholamines as well as of pituitary hormones, probably reflecting a direct stimulation of neuroendocrine centers in the CNS by impulses from motor centers. As oxygen uptake and blood lactate were identical with and without curarization in the first work period, the higher hormonal response in the former experiment was probably not due to a higher input of afferent impulses from working muscles to neuroendocrine centers. The finding of identical values of perceived exertion and hormonal responses in Cu and C experiments in the second work period was in accordance with a direct role of central command in the regulation of hormonal response to exercise. Also the metabolic data agreed with a direct stimulation of autonomic neuroendocrine activity by central command during exercise. In the first work period lipid mobilization as judged from concentrations of glycerol and FFA in plasma varied in parallel with motor center activity. Glucose production was enhanced in tubocurarine experiments as seen from the findings that the initial increase in glucose production during exercise was higher in these than in control experiments, and that the plasma glucose increased only in the former experiments. The exercise-induced increase in glucose production preceding a rise in glucose disappearance and resulting in an increase in plasma glucose has previously been demonstrated in rats (Sonne & Galbo, 1985) as well as in physically well trained humans (Kjaer et al., 1986). Feed forward control of glucose production is also strongly suggested by the recent finding that at high work loads glucose utilization may decrease in the face of increasing muscular glucose uptake (Katz et al., 1986).

Evidently, to test the validity of the hypothesis that central command is directly involved in the regulation of exercise metabolism it is crucial to study paralyzed animals in which fictive locomotion is developed spontaneously or induced by electrical or chemical stimulation of motor centers in the brain (Eldridge et al., 1985). However, from the present study in humans it is concluded that activity in motor centers may directly elicit symphatoadrenal responses as well as pituitary hormonal secretion and, in turn, substrate mobilization during dynamic exercise.

Acknowledgments

The study was supported by Danish Medical and Sports Research Council, P. Carl Petersen Foundation, and the NOVO Foundation.

References

Eldridge, F.L., Millhorn, E.D., Kiley, J.P., & Waldrop, G. (1985). Stimulation by central command of locomotion, respiration and circulation during exercise. *Respiration Physiol.*, **59**, 313-337.

Galbo, H. (1983). *Hormonal and metabolic adaptation to exercise.* Georg Thieme Verlag, Stuttgart, New York.

Katz, A., Broberg, S., Sahlin, K., & Wahren, J. (1986). Leg glucose uptake during maximal exercise in man. *Am. J. Physiol.,* **251**, E65-E70.

Kjaer, M., Farrel, P.A., Christensen, N.J., & Galbo, H. (1986). Increased epinephrine response and inaccurate glucose regulation in exercising athletes. *J. Appl. Physiol.,* **61**, 1693-1700.

Sonne, B., & Galbo, H. (1985). Carbohydrate metabolism during and after exercise in rats: Studies with radio glucose. *J. Appl. Physiol.,* **59**, 1627-1639.

The Hypothalmic and Neurohypophysial Vasopressin and Oxytocin Content in Immobilized or Cold-Exposed Rats

S. Olczak, A. Lewandowska, and J. Guzek

Department of Pathophysiology, School of Medicine, Łódź, Poland

Immobilization or exposure to cold (2-5 °C) were applied to male albino rats of the Wistar strain. The animals were killed after 24 h and the hypothalmic and neurohypophysial vasopressin and oxytocin contents were bioassayed. Stress due to immobilization was followed by diminution of vasopressin and oxytocin contents both in the hypothalamus and neurohypophysis. In rats exposed to cold the hypothalamic and neurohypophysial vasopressor and oxytocic activities were increased. It is supposed that both vasopressinergic and oxytocinergic neurones are involved in the mechanisms of stress. The response of these neurones seems to be dependent on the kind of stressor (Table 1).

Table 1 The Hypothalamic and Neurohypophysial Vasopressor and Oxytocic Activities in Stressed Rats

Group of animals	Vasopressor activity		Oxytocic activity	
	Hypothalamus	Neurohypophysis	Hypothalamus	Neurohypophysis
a - controls	41.6 ± 1.9	574 ± 38.8	45.7 ± 1.7	584 ± 17.6
b - animals deprived of food and water	38.9 ± 2.1	471 ± 15.4	36.8 ± 2.4	506 ± 16.7
c - animals exposed to cold	41.3 ± 1.3	523 ± 15.7	52.0 ± 1.7	519 ± 23.4
d - animals immobilized	26.9 ± 1.7	396 ± 16.6	23.4 ± 1.6	377 ± 14.6
Significance as estimated by Student's t test:				
a versus b	NS	$p < .025$	$p < .01$	$p < .005$
b versus c	NS	$p < .05$	$p < .001$	NS
b versus d	$p < .001$	$p < .005$	$p < .001$	$p < .001$

Note. NS = not significant; mU per whole hypothalamus or neurohypophysis; mean $\pm$ *SEM*.

Effects of Exhausting Physical Exercise on Plasma Insulin Levels in Young Cyclists

R. Stupnicki and A. Wiśniewska

Institute of Sport, Warsaw, Poland

Physical exercise of moderate intensity (approx. 50% $\dot{V}O_2$max) decreases plasma insulin levels in nontrained individuals, the degree of this decrease depending on the intensity and duration of exercise. Moreover, untrained individuals show greater decrease after the exercise, as compared with the trained ones. The aim of this work was to study changes in plasma glucose and insulin levels as affected by exercise of increasing intensity performed by 35 young cyclists (16-18 yrs of age), until exhaustion. Cycloergometer exercise of varying length (12-45 min) was applied. Blood sampling took place before exercise, and 2 and 15 min after the exercise was terminated. This study was repeated three times over the year. The increase of plasma glucose level after the exercise was similar in all studied subjects. Two min after the exercise, a decrease in insulin level was observed in 60% of studied subjects, while in the remaining 40% there was an increase. A pattern of the response was significantly characteristic for a given individual. This nonuniformity of insulin response to exercise could have resulted from different reactivity of pancreatic beta-cells to exercise-induced hyperglycemia and from different sensitivity of peripheral tissues to insulin.

Part V

Thermoregulation and Body Temperature Responses to Exercise

On the Location and Nature of Central Thermosensitive Structures in Homeotherms

C. Jessen

Physiologisches Institut der Universitaet, Giessen, F.R.G.

Thermosensitive elements in the skin and the body core of homeotherms generate afferent temperature signals the central integration of which provides the regulated variable of the thermoregulatory system and the efferent commands to effector mechanisms producing or dissipating heat. Previous equations describing the relationships between skin and core temperatures on one hand, and production or dissipation of heat on the other, were mostly derived from experiments in humans (e.g., Stolwijk & Hardy, 1966), which limited the extent to which skin and core temperatures could be dissociated. Therefore, a new attempt was undertaken to make skin and core temperatures truly independent variables: Conscious goats were immersed in a water bath to clamp skin temperature at predetermined levels in the range of 32° to 44 °C, while core temperature was altered between 35° and 42 °C by means of heat exchangers acting on arterial blood temperature (Nagel et al., 1986). The left side of Figure 1 comprises the results of 20 experiments in a single animal. The heavy central line joins all combinations of skin and core temperatures, in which heat production (META < 2.0 W/kg) and respiratory evaporative heat loss (REHL < 0.3 W/kg) were at resting levels. The slope of this line is indicative of the relative inputs provided by skin and core temperatures: The effect of a 12 °C change in skin temperature was balanced by a 1.3 °C change in core temperature. The broken contour lines for higher levels of heat production and heat loss confirm this pattern: The response per unit change of core temperature by far exceeded that of a change of skin temperature.

Another aspect of Figure 1 is that even at a skin temperature of 44 °C, a large increase in heat production due to shivering could be observed when core temperature was sufficiently low. This finding contradicts previous observations in humans (Benzinger, 1969) and animals (Cabanac, 1970), which were extrapolated to indicate that the control of effector responses conforms to a multiplicative model of interaction. Our experiments strongly suggest an additive type of interaction of skin and core temperature signals in control of thermoregulatory effector systems.

The contour lines on the right side of Figure 1 were derived from multiple linear regressions on data of the left side of the figure: $META = 10.04 - 1.85 \, (1.38^{(T_{core} - 34)}) + 0.36$ $(44.2 - T_{skin})$; $R = 0.81$; $n = 1630$. $REHL = -1.01 + 0.45 \, (1.29^{(T_{core} - 34)}) - 0.06$ $(44.2 - T_{skin})$; $R = 0.79$; $n = 885$. The type of equation assumes that the afferent input to the controlling system consists of two counteracting fractions: cold signals linearly related to skin temperature and warm signals that increase exponentially with core temperature. What evidence is available to support the second assumption, which gave reason to transform the core temperature values in exponential terms?

In a recent study on conscious goats, experiments were made to determine the relationship between core temperature and core temperature signals (Jessen & Feistkorn, 1984). For this purpose goats were instrumented to permit independent control of head and trunk temperatures. Since both parts of the body core are known to provide approximately equal fractions of the integrated core temperature signal, large thermal gradients between head

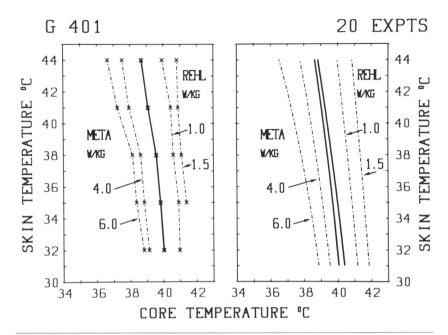

Figure 1. Skin temperature and core temperature in control of heat production (META) and respiratory evaporative heat loss (REHL). The heavy line on the left joins all temperature combinations in which heat production and heat loss were simultaneously at resting levels. Right side: Lines derived from multiple regressions on raw data of left side. The two heavy lines indicate levels of 2 W/kg (META) and 0.5 W/kg (REHL), which are at or close to resting values. Data from Nagel et al. (1986).

and trunk of more than 6 °C were created in order to determine the pattern of combinations of both inputs, which resulted in equal levels of heat production and heat loss, respectively. The shape of the resulting contour lines revealed that the input generated per unit of either head or trunk temperatures increased with higher levels of temperature.

Consequently, if META or REHL were plotted versus head or trunk temperatures at constant levels of the other input, the effector responses were found to be nonlinearly related to temperature, that is, showing increasing slopes with increasing temperature (Figure 2). One conceivable explanation is that the temperature–response curve of core sensors of temperature resembles that of warm receptors. Another interpretation would argue that the relationship between temperature and signal generation is linear, while any nonlinearities are caused by an unspecific thermosensitivity of signal transmission in the central nervous system (Simon et al., 1986). Present evidence does not permit to distinguish between these possibilities.

As to the location of central thermosensitive structures, evidence has been accumulating in recent years that the hypothalamus is not the only thermosensitive site within the body core. The lower brain stem, medulla, and spinal cord contain thermosensitive elements, the inputs of which into the central regulator have been documented both in the conscious animal and in studies involving single neuron recordings (see Jessen, 1985).

In the past it has been frequently postulated that muscle thermoreceptors participate in control of body temperature (Stolwijk & Hardy, 1966; Werner, 1980). However, until recently only circumstantial evidence has been available in favor of or against the existence

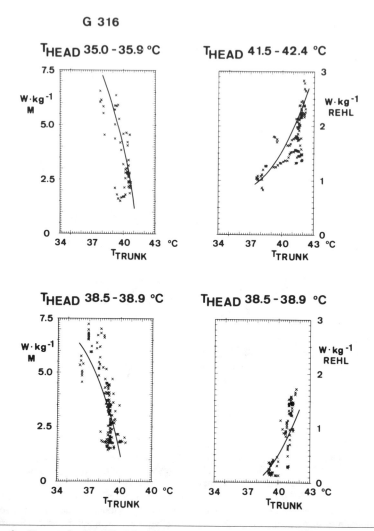

Figure 2. Heat production (M) and respiratory evaporative heat loss (REHL) versus trunk temperature for selected ranges of head temperature. Note that M and REHL varied in parallel with trunk temperature at constant levels of head (i.e., brain and hypothalamic) temperature. Data from Jessen and Feistkorn (1984).

and action of muscle thermoreceptors. In 1983 a study was performed to isolate a fraction of the total musculature thermally and to correlate thermal responses of a conscious animal with experimentally induced alterations of temperature in these muscles. Stainless steel thermodes of 10-12 mm diameter and 100-150 mm length chronically implanted into the marrow spaces of both humeri and femora, all of which have in goats wide cavities and thin walls (Jessen et al., 1983). Perfusing the thermodes with water of 0 °C altered the temperature of the deep muscle layers surrounding the bones by several degrees C. The animals were further equipped with intravascular heat exchangers which served to keep general body temperature constant during periods of leg cooling (Jessen, 1981).

Figure 3 shows a standard experiment in a hot and dry environment. From the 30th to the 60th minute all four upper limbs were cooled while general body core temperature (T_{paor}) was maintained constant. This caused panting, as quantified by the respiratory evaporative heat loss (REHL), to decrease from 2.2 to 1.9 W/kg. This small but significant response was regularly observed and indicates a local effect of the cooling on deep thermosensitive elements in the legs themselves and a neural afferent transmission of temperature signals to the central regulator of body temperature.

Concerning the nature of the neural afferents involved in mediating the response to leg cooling, a number of pertinent studies have been published (see Mitchell & Schmidt, 1983). Any muscle nerve contains many more fine afferents (groups III and IV) than the well known large afferent units of groups I and II, which serve muscle spindles and Golgi organs. When these fine afferents were tested for temperature sensitivity, it turned out that approximately 50% of all units under investigation responded to non-noxious thermal stimuli in the range of 24-44 °C (Hertel et al., 1976; Mense & Meyer, 1985). In fact, many of these units behaved like cold or warm receptors in the skin, and might well present the

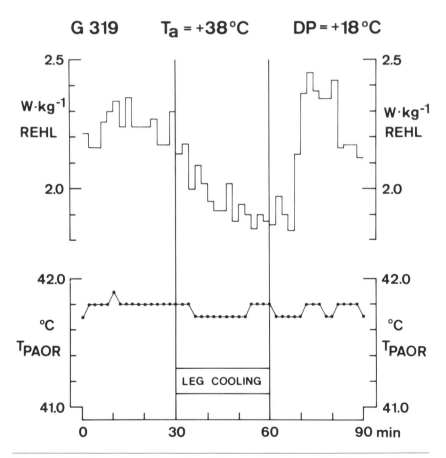

Figure 3. Selective cooling of the muscles of the upper limbs (leg cooling) by means of thermodes implanted in the marrow spaces of both humeri and femora reduces the heat loss response to high body temperature. Data from Jessen et al. (1983).

nervous correlate to the thermoregulatory responses to heating or cooling the skeletal muscle in the conscious goat.

The afferent neurons signaling muscle temperature could also be of relevance to explaining the observation that the level of muscle temperature during exercise correlates well with exhaustion. The link between these two phenomena is often seen in a local effect of temperature on muscle metabolism and has been well demonstrated in a recent series of experiments by Kozłowski et al. (1985).

Figure 4 is compiled from their data. Eleven dogs ran twice on a treadmill to exhaustion, with speeds adjusted to their body size. In the first experiment the dogs were externally cooled by carrying ice bags, while the second experiment served as a control. External cooling decreased the rise in muscle temperature by 1 °C and increased work performance time from 57 to 83 min. In the noncooled condition needle biopsies taken from the m. vastus lateralis showed an average lactate concentration of 85 mmol/kg dry weight and a muscle glycogen content of 150 mmol/kg.

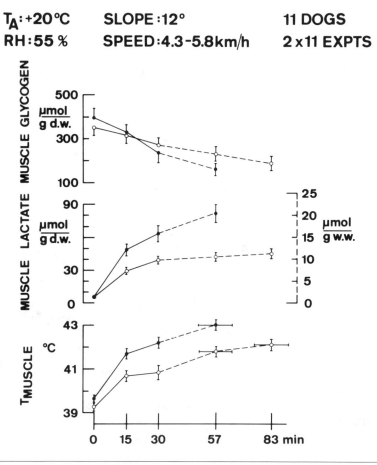

Figure 4. Effects of body temperature on muscle metabolism in exercising dogs. Body temperature was either free running (filled circles), or increasing at a reduced rate due to external cooling (open circles). Muscle temperature and needle biopsies were taken from the m. vastus lateralis. Data from Kozlowski et al. (1985).

The data are taken to indicate that hyperthermia accelerates glycolysis, which might exert an adverse effect on muscle metabolism and is relevant to the thermal limits of endurance. A complementary view is that neural afferents from the exercising muscle, stimulated by temperature and the local biochemical environment, might contribute to the central generation of a signal enforcing the cessation of exercise. Muscle afferents have been shown to be highly sensitive to local concentrations of potassium and lactate (Thimm & Tibes, 1978). In Kozłowski's experiments, muscle lactate concentration at a muscle temperature of 43 °C was twice as large as at a muscle temperature of 42 °C, and it appears conceivable that the effect of lactate on neural afferents has acted in parallel with the local effects on metabolism to determine that level of muscle temperature beyond which exercise could not be continued.

Acknowledgments

Supported by DFG Je 57/8. The secretarial work of Mrs. D. Felde is appreciated.

References

Benzinger, T.H. (1969). Heat regulation: Homeostasis of central temperature in man. *Physiological Reviews,* **49**, 671-759.

Cabanac, M. (1970). Interaction of cold and warm temperature signals in the brain stem. In J.D. Hardy, A.P. Gagge, & J.A.J. Stolwijk (Eds.), *Physiological and behavioral temperature regulation.* Springfield, Thomas, 549-561.

Hertel, H.C., Howaldt, B., & Mense, S. (1976). Responses of group IV and group III muscle afferents to thermal stimuli. *Brain Research,* **113**, 201-205.

Jessen, C. (1981). Independent clamps of peripheral and central temperatures and their effects on heat production in the goat. *Journal of Physiology (London),* **311**, 11-21.

Jessen, C. (1985). Thermal afferents in the control of body temperature. *Pharmacology and Therapeutics,* **28**, 107-134.

Jessen, C., Feistkorn, G., & Nagel, A. (1983). Temperature sensitivity of skeletal muscle in the conscious goat. *Journal of Applied Physiology,* **54**, 880-886.

Jessen, C. & Feistkorn, G. (1984). Some characteristics of core temperature signals in the conscious goat. *American Journal of Physiology,* **247**, R 456-R 464.

Kozłowski, S., Brzezinska, Z., Kruk, B. Kaciuba-Uścilko, H., Greenleaf, J.E., & Nazar, K. (1985). Exercise hyperthermia as a factor limiting physical performance: Temperature effect on muscle metabolism. *Journal of Applied Physiology,* **59**, 766-773.

Mense, S., & Meyer, H. (1985). Different types of slowly conducting afferent units in cat skeletal muscle and tendon. *Journal of Physiology (London),* **363**, 403-418.

Mitchell, J.M., & Schmidt, R.F. (1983). Cardiovascular reflex control by afferent fibers from skeletal muscle receptors. In J.T. Shepherd & F.M. Abboud (Eds.), *Handbook of physiology. The cardiovascular system, Vol III, Part 2.* American Physiological Society, Bethesda, MD, 623-658.

Nagel, A., Herold, W., Roos, R., & Jessen, C. (1986). Skin and core temperatures as determinants of heat production and heat loss in the goat. *Pfluegers Archives,* **406**, 600-607.

Simon, E., Pierau, F.-K., Taylor, D.C.M. (1986). Central and peripheral thermal control of effectors in homeothermic temperature regulation. *Physiological Reviews,* **66**, 235-300.

Stolwijk, J.A.J., & Hardy, J.D. (1966). Temperature regulation in man—A theoretical study. *Pfluegers Archives,* **291**, 129-162.

Werner, J. (1980). The concept of regulation for human body temperature. *Journal of Thermal Biology,* **5**, 75-82.

RESEARCH NOTES

Thermoregulatory Adaptation to Exercise in the Course of Endurance Training

J. Smorawiński, R. Grucza, and S. Kozłowski
Department of Sports Medicine, Academy of Physical Education, Poznań and Department of Applied Physiology, Medical Research Centre, Polish Academy of Sciences, Warsaw, Poland

There is a controversy in the literature concerning mechanisms of thermal and exercise adaptation to heat. The controversy concerns mainly the mechanism of sweating response during exercise in heat-acclimated and physically trained men. Strydom et al. (1966) suggested that physical training cannot replace the true heat-acclimation procedure since no changes in the sweating rate occur in exercising trained men. On the other hand, Baum et al. (1976) reported a significant decrease in the sweating threshold in trained men, concluding that endurance training produces modifications in the sweating mechanism which are not different from those produced by heat acclimation. This conclusion is opposite to the results presented by Shvartz et al. (1974), who demonstrated a decrease in sweating rate in response to exercise during the training program in temperate climate.

The aim of the present work was, therefore, to elucidate the influence of endurance training on thermoregulatory responses to exercise performed by men under thermoneutral conditions. Special attention was paid to possible changes in the sweating dynamics in the exercising subjects.

Material and Methods

Twenty-eight healthy men aged 21 ± 1 years participated in this study. The subjects underwent a 3-month training program consisting of 1 h running for 3 days a week, everyday calisthenics followed by 3 km jogging plus 2 h basketball playing once a week. Before, after, and every month of the training period the subjects performed 60-min bicycle ergometer exercise with an intensity of 50% $\dot{V}O_2$max in thermoneutral environment (ambient and wall temp. 22 °C, relative air humidity 45%).

Maximal oxygen uptake ($\dot{V}O_2$max) was measured directly the day before each exercise test. During each exercise test heart rate (HR) was continuously monitored by ECG, and the metabolic heat production was calculated from O_2 uptake and CO_2 elimination measurements (Spirolit 2 VEB Junkalor Dessau). Cutaneous temperatures on chest, arm, and thigh were measured by teleinfrared thermometer (Era, Poznań). Mean skin temperature was calculated according to the formula $\bar{T}_{sk} = 0.50\ T_{chest} + 0.36\ T_{thigh} + 0.14\ T_{arm}$.

Auditory canal temperature (T_{ac}) was measured with a zerogradient aural thermometer (Muirhead, 8151.1). An increase in mean body temperature was calculated as follows: $\Delta\bar{T}_b = 0.8\ \Delta T_{ac} + 0.2\ \Delta T_{sk}$. Dynamics of sweating was estimated based on the changes in electrical skin resistance (ESR) and measured using disposable unpolarized ECG electrodes fixed to the skin of the sternal area (Grucza, 1983). It was characterized by a delay time (T_d), time constant (τ), and intertia time (T_i)—the sum of delay and time constant.

Results

1. Maximal oxygen uptake ($\dot{V}O_2$max) increased in the course of training from 3.16 ± 0.34 to 3.72 ± 0.34 L • min^{-1}, $p < .001$, with the most pronounced changes (0.40 L • min^{-1}) during the first month. Heart rate (HR) measured at rest differed significantly from the control value only after the third month of training (ΔHr, 8 beats • min^{-1}, $p < .001$).

2. Elevations in the auditory canal temperature (ΔT_{ac}) during exercise were progressively lowered with the duration of training. The unchanged value of $\Delta\bar{T}_b$ with decreasing ΔT_{ac} was a result of higher mean skin temperature response to exercise at the end of training.

3. Exercise-induced body weight loss Δ_w increased gradually in the course of training from 505 ± 131 to 609 ± 93 g ($p < .005$). A delay in the onset of sweating was significantly reduced after the training with the time constant of the reaction decreasing from 9.3 ± 4.3 to 4.9 ± 1.6 min ($p < .001$).

4. There was a relationship between the exercise-induced increase in the auditory canal temperature (ΔT_{ac}), body weight loss (Δ_w), and the inertia time of sweating. The faster sweating response to exercise that developed during endurance training enabled greater sweat loss and, consequently, greater heat dissipation in the exercising men, thus attenuating an increase in body temperature.

Discussion

The endurance training caused an increase in the maximal aerobic capacity of the subjects by 17.7%. This value corresponds well to the $\dot{V}O_2$max increases reported after different programs of training (Ekblom et al., 1968). The finding that the main changes in $\dot{V}O_2$max appeared already after one month of training suggests that significant changes in $\dot{V}O_2$max can develop within a few weeks if the training stimulus is appropriately high and constant.

Faster triggering of sweating resulting in the significant attenuation of hyperthermia, expressed as ΔT_{ac}, during exercise developed gradually in the time course of training despite the slow increase of $\dot{V}O_2$max during the last two months. Frequently repeated exercise with a relatively high intensity in the course of endurance training can adapt men to heat. It seems likely that the main differences between acclimation to exogenous heat (heat exposure) and to endogenous heat (exercise) consist in the lack of peripheral thermoreceptor activation and facilitation of heat transport to body surface in the latter case. Endogenous heat produced during physical exercise obviously stimulates thermoregulatory mechanisms either directly or via muscle and other internal thermoreceptors.

The results presented show that endurance training causes an increase in dynamics of sweating by shortening the inertia time of this response to exercise. This effect, known as a downward shift of sweating threshold (Baum et al., 1976) or reduction in the central nervous system point of zero sweating drive (Nadel et al., 1974), is generally connected with lower body temperatures in exercising trained men. Considering the sweating threshold, however, one should take into account that sweating reaction in response to exercise usually appears before noticeable increase in tympanic, rectal, muscle, or skin temperatures (Beaumont & Bullard, 1963; Saltin et al., 1970). According to our results the delay in onset of sweating at the beginning of exercise was shortened from 4 min before to 0.8 min after the training and no significant differences in T_{ac} were observed during this period of exercise. Since the lag of sweating may be due to the filling of the duct of the gland with sweat and to its further transport to the skin surface (Bullard, 1971) it is suggested that endurance training may improve this mechanism as a part of overall physiological adaptation to exercise.

Conclusion

This study demonstrated that endurance training results in an improvement of thermo-regulatory efficiency manifested by earlier onset of sweating response, with a subsequent attenuation of exercise hyperthermia.

References

Baum, E., Brück, K., & Schwennicke, H.P. (1976). Adaptative modifications in the thermo-regulatory system of long-distance runners. *J. Appl. Physiol.*, **40**, 404-410.

Beaumont, W., & Bullard, R.W. (1963). Sweating: The rapid response to muscular work. *Science*, **141**, 643-646.

Bullard, R.W. (1971). Studies on human sweat gland duct filling and skin hydration. *J. Physiol. Paris*, **63**, 218-221.

Ekblom, B., Åstrand, P.O., Saltin, B., Stenberg, J., & Wallström, B. (1968). Effect of training on circulatory response to exercise. *J. Appl. Physiol.*, **24**, 518-528.

Gisolfi, C., & Robinson, S. (1969). Relations between physical training, acclimatization, and heat tolerance. *J. Appl. Physiol.*, **26**, 530-534.

Grucza, R. (1983). Body heat balance in man subjected to endogenous and exogenous heat load. *Eur. J. Appl. Physiol.*, **51**, 419-433.

Hanson, J.S., Tabakin, B.S., Levy, A.M., & Nedde, W. (1968). Long term physical training and cardiovascular dynamics in middle-aged men. *Circulation*, **38**, 783-799.

Hickson, R.C., Bonze, H.A., & Holloszy, J.O. (1977). Linear increase in aerobic power induced by a strenuous program of endurance exercise. *J. Appl. Physiol.: Respirat. Environ. Exercise Physiol.*, **42**, 372-376.

Knuttgen, H.G., Nordesjö, L.-O., Ollander, B., & Saltin, B. (1973). Physical conditioning through interval training with young male adults. *Med. Sci. Sports*, **5**, 220-226.

Nadel, E.R., Pandolf, K.B., Roberts, M.F., & Stolwijk, J.A.J. (1974). Mechanisms of thermal acclimation to exercise and heat. *J. Appl. Physiol.*, **37**, 515-520.

Piwonka, R.W., Robinson, S., Gay, V.L., & Manalis, R.S. (1965). Preacclimation of men to heat by training. *J. Appl. Physiol.*, **20**, 379-384.

Piwonka, R.W., & Robinson, S. (1967). Acclimatization of highly trained men to work in severe heat. *J. Appl. Physiol.*, **20**, 9-12.

Pollock, M.L. (1973). The quantification of endurance training program. In J.H. Wilmore (Ed.), *Exercise and Sport Science Reviews*. New York, Academic Press, vol. 1, 155-188.

Saltin, B., Gagge, A.P., & Stolwijk, J.A.J. (1970). Body temperatures and sweating during thermal transients caused by exercise. *J. Appl. Physiol.*, **28**, 318-327.

Shvartz, E., Magazanik, A., & Glick, Z. (1974). Thermal responses during training in a temperate climate. *J. Appl. Physiol.*, **36**, 572-576.

Strydom, N.B., Wyndham, C.H., Williams, C.G., Morrison, J.F., Bredell, G.A.G., Benade, A.J.S., & Rahden van, M. (1966). Acclimatization to humid heat and the role of physical conditioning. *J. Appl. Physiol.*, **21**, 636-642.

Wilmore, J.H., Royce, J., Girandola, R.N., Katch, F.I., & Katch, V.L. (1970). Physiological alterations resulting from a 10 week program of jogging. *Med. Sci. Sports*, **2**, 7-17.

The Effect of Warming Up on Thermoregulatory Responses to Incremental Exercise and on the Anaerobic Threshold in Men

J. Chwalbińska-Moneta and O. Hänninen

Department of Applied Physiology, Medical Research Centre, Polish Academy of Sciences, Warsaw, Poland and Department of Physiology, University of Kuopio, Finland

The influence of 10 min of warming up at 40% $\dot{V}O_2$max on thermal, circulatory, and metabolic responses to an incremental exercise until exhaustion as well as on the anaerobic threshold at the blood lactate of 4 mmol $\cdot$ L^{-1} (AT) and the individual anaerobic threshold (IAT) was investigated in 8 cross-country skiers under thermoneutral conditions. During exercise preceded by warming up, the mean skin temperature ($\bar{T}_{sk}$) and external auditory canal temperature (T_{ac}) did not change significantly in contrast to exercise without warming up, producing a rise in both $\bar{T}_{sk}$ and T_{ac} (by approx. 1.2 °C and 1.1 °C, respectively). Warming up did not alter the course of the rectal temperature changes during exercise.

With warming up, skin humidity, reflecting the rate of sweating, rose immediately after the beginning of exercise, whereas the onset of sweating without warming up appeared much later (at higher work intensities). Warming up did not change the circulatory and ventilatory responses to incremental exercise and the oxygen uptake ($\dot{V}O_2$) either at submaximal or maximal work loads. With warming up a significant increase was found in the threshold work load both at the AT and the IAT as well as in the threshold $\dot{V}O_2$ and heart rate at the IAT. The data demonstrated that warming up has an advantageous effect on the efficiency of thermoregulation in endurance-trained athletes, producing an early sweating response to the incremental exercise that results in attenuation of hyperthermia. An increase in the anaerobic threshold during incremental exercise preceded by warning up may indicate an enhancement of the endurance capacity subsequent to warming up.

How to Improve the Exercise Thermoregulatory Functions

R. Kubica, B. Wilk, J. Stokłosa, and A. Żuchowicz

Department of Physiology and Sport Medicine, Academy of Physical Education, Kraków, Poland

This study was undertaken to compare the effects of two physical training programs accomplished in temperate and hot environments on thermoregulatory responses to exercise. Duration of a particular training exercise session was 90 min in temperate, and it was individually differentiated in the hot environment. The latter depended upon the time necessary to increase rectal temperature (T_{re}) to the level similar to that achieved during 90-min exertion at room temperature. As a consequence this time varied from 20 to 40 min. This experimental approach was a result of a hypothesis that the same thermal stimulus, that is, an increase in T_{re} of the same order as after exercise training at room temperature, will evoke similar training-induced effects on thermoregulatory responses. If it is true, the achievement of similar improvement of thermoregulatory mechanisms in thermal-exercise training will be possible owing to the shorter exercise sessions saving the body energy stores.

The male physical education students participated in this study. Physical training performed in the hot environment (33 °C $\pm$ 1 °C, 50% of relative humidity) did not affect either the level of maximum oxygen uptake or the average oxygen uptake during the prolonged 90-min exercise test executed in temperate environment (21 °C $\pm$ 1 °C, 50% $\pm$ 5% of relative humidity). In spite of the lack of any changes in metabolic reactions to exercise the improvement of thermoregulatory responses could be observed. It was expressed by a lower level and a smaller increase of rectal temperature (ΔT_{re}) and heart rate (ΔHR) as well as a greater decrease in the mean skin temperature ($\Delta \bar{T}_{sk}$) at the end of prolonged 90-min exercise on bicycle ergometer.

Behavioral Thermoregulatory Responses in Obese and Control Women

B. Zahorska-Markiewicz

Department of Physiology, Institute of Occupational Medicine, Sosnowiec, Poland

There are studies suggesting that the thermoregulation "set point" can be estimated in human subjects on the basis of preference of locally applied thermal stimuli. The aim of this study was to determine whether obese subjects differ from normal weight or lean controls in thermal preference. Twenty-two obese women aged 16 to 52 years with over-weight ranging from 41 to 130% (mean 73.8) participated in this study. Twenty normal weight (mean 55 kg) and 10 lean women (mean 49.4 kg) of similar age served as a control group. The subjects were immersed in a water bath at 37 °C. Their oral temperature (T_o) was measured. The subject's left hand was periodically immersed for 30 s in a small tank filled with water of temperature varying between 20 and 45 °C. The subjects were asked to indicate the most pleasant temperature. The oral temperature in the obese women (36.9 ± 0.3 °C) was lower ($p < .001$) than that in controls (37.3 ± 0.2 °C). The control women rated hand immersion in water of 40 to 45 °C as very pleasant, and that of 20 °C as very unpleasant. The majority of obese women indicated water temperature 20 to 35 °C as preferable. The shift in the temperature preference toward lower values in the obese women was statistically significant ($p < .01$). In conclusion, the data indicate that in the simple obesity thermogenesis is reduced, which results in lowering of core body temperature. Moreover, it seems likely that in obese women the thermoregulatory "set-point" is shifted toward lower values.

Part VI
Clinical Aspects of Physical Activity

RESEARCH NOTES

Interrelationships Between Age, Obesity, Pattern of Fat Distribution, Physical Fitness, and Metabolic Risk Factors for Coronary Artery Disease

A.W. Ziemba, J. Fleg, and R. Andres

Department of Applied Physiology, Medical Research Centre, Polish Academy of Sciences, Warsaw, Poland and Gerontology Research Center, National Institute on Aging, National Institutes of Health, Baltimore, MD, U.S.A.

Risk factors for Coronary Artery Disease (CAD) include biological, metabolic, cardiovascular factors, and also certain living habits. Some of these factors cannot be modified. They include such biological variables as age, male sex, and family history of CAD. Potentially modifiable risk factors include such metabolic variables as hyperlipidemia, hyperglycemia, and the major cardiovascular risk factor—hypertension. Overweight is known to be associated with all of these factors. More recently the pattern of fat distribution has been considered as an important contributory variable. Physical fitness interacts with all these variables and may have an independent effect on development of CAD as well. A decline in physical fitness and an increase in body adiposity are parallel to human aging. Thus, relationships between aging, obesity, body fat distribution, physical fitness, and other coronary risk factors are complex and interdependent (Figure 1). These interrelationships were not taken into account in a number of studies concentrating on the beneficial aspects of physical fitness. The purpose of the present study was to evaluate the contribution of age, obesity, and working capacity on some metabolic changes considered as risk factors for CAD.

Material and Methods

The data were obtained from 278 male volunteers, participants of the Baltimore Longitudinal Study on Aging (BLSA). The subjects' age was 22 to 87 yrs. Subjects with diseases or on medication known to influence glucose tolerance were excluded form the analyses. The following variables were taken into account in the present study: age; index of overweight—Body Mass Index, $BMI = w \cdot h^{-2}$ (w = weight in kg, h = height in m); index of fat distribution—waist girth to hip girth ratio WHR (W = minimal circumferences of abdomen, H = circumference of buttock at maximal gluteal protuberance); physical fitness—maximal oxygen uptake ($\dot{V}O_2max$); and metabolic variables—fasting plasma glucose (FPG), plasma glucose concentration at 2 h after oral glucose load of 40 g/m² (oral glucose

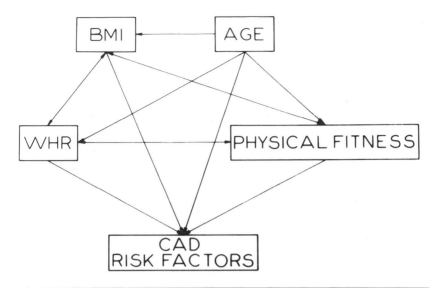

Figure 1. The interrelationships between age, body mass index (BMI), waist/hip ratio (WHR), physical fitness, and coronary artery disease risk factors.

tolerance test, OGTT), total serum cholesterol, HDL, and LDL levels, HDL/HDL ratio and plasma triglyceride (TG) concentration. Both simple bivariate regression and multivariate statistical techniques were applied to assess relationships between independent variables (age, BMI, WHR, $\dot{V}O_2$max) and metabolic indices designed as dependent variables.

Results

The simple regression analysis showed that each of the dependent variables was closely related to age, BMI, WHR, and $\dot{V}O_2$max. Correlations between the dependent variables were also ascertained. As it is shown on Figure 2 the aerobic capacity is decreasing with age and with increasing BMI. The equation for a dependent variable calculated by the multiple regression analysis is as follows: Dependent variable = Intercept + a Age + b BMI + c WHR + d $\dot{V}O_2$max. The results of this analysis and r values are summarized in Table 1.

As it is shown in Table 1, when the multiple regression analysis was applied it was demonstrated that both age and BMI influence significantly the fasting glucose level, glucose concentration 2 h after glucose load and total cholesterol, while $\dot{V}O_2$max was a dominant factor determining blood lipoproteins HDL, LDL, and HDL/LDL ratio. WHR affected significantly only the plasma TG (expressed as its log) and glucose concentration in the OGTT. In spite of the lack of the direct impact of physical working capacity on fasting level of blood glucose, the response to OGTT, total cholesterol, and TG concentration it seems likely that physical fitness can exert its effects on carbohydrate metabolism and some indices of lipid metabolism indirectly by influencing body weight, so that it loses its strong independent significance on multivariate analysis. There is, however, still another possibility: Population studies that include a large number of very highly active and well fit individuals may show significant fitness effects not demonstrated in this population.

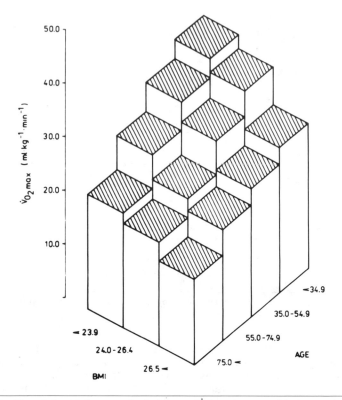

Figure 2.   The relationship between physical fitness (V̇O₂max), age, and body mass index (BMI).

Table 1   Results of the Multiple Regression Analysis

Dependent variables	Intercept	Age (a)	BMI (b)	WHR (c)	V̇O₂max (d)	r
FPG	65.3	0.138**	0.928**	—	—	0.433
OGTT	−80.07	0.006**	2.26*	193.3*	—	0.520
TG	0.5112	—	0.15	1.256	—	0.480
CHOL	101.77	0.455*	2.489*	—	—	0.293
HDL	24.388	0.123*	—	—	0.241*	0.220
LDL	150.86	—	—	—	−0.791**	0.270
LDL/HDL	4.279	—	—	—	−0.028	0.280

Note. a, b, c, d are the coefficients of the regression; r = correlation coefficient; *$p < .01$. **$p < .001$.

An Attempt to Modify the Preventive and Rehabilitative Training Programs Based on Exercise-Induced Haemostatic Changes

W. Drygas and L. Röcker

Department of Sports Medicine, Medical Academy, Lódź, Poland and Institut für Leistungsmedizin, Freie Universität, Berlin, West Germany

There is extensive evidence that disorders in blood platelet function, coagulation, and fibrinolysis may play a crucial role in the pathogenesis of atherogenesis and sudden fatalities. In spite of currently prevalent opinion that regular exercise has long-term beneficial effects on health, it must be remembered that a high proportion of myocardial infarctions, reinfarctions, and cardiac arrests continue to occur during physical activity (Jokl, 1975; Samek et al., 1982; Shephard, 1984; Wybitul et al., 1983). Several studies have shown that strenuous exercise may influence blood platelet, intrinsic coagulation pathway, and fibrinolysis. Intracoronary occlusions have been found in some cases of myocardial infarction and in sudden cardiac deaths following strenuous physical exertion (Jokl, 1975; Wybitul et al., 1983). Nevertheless, exercise prescriptions presented in many books and reviews are based traditionally on aerobic capacity changes due to the exercise. In this paper we have summarized some data from our experimental studies, performed in 1983-1986, concerning effects of exercise on the haemostatic system in healthy untrained men aged 16 to 62 years, recreational and competitive sportsmen, and post-infarction patients (Drygas et al., 1986; Drygas, in press; Röcker et al., 1984; Röcker et al., 1986).

Methods

Several exercise tests varying with regard to the form, duration, and intensity have been applied. Apart from routine coagulation tests (platelet counts, PTT, prothrombin time, thrombin and reptilase time, fibrinogen, euglobulin lysis time), we have carried out some specific tests measuring platelet activity (β-tromboglobulin, platelet factor 4, circulate platelets aggregates), thrombin activity (fibrinopeptide A), fibrin degradation products and coagulation, and fibrinolysis inhibitors. Materials and methods have been described in detail elsewhere (Drygas, in press; Röcker et al., 1984; Röcker et al., 1986).

Results and Discussion

From the results we have obtained it appears that intensive exercises connected with marked acidosis as well as strenuous prolonged exercise may adversely affect the haemostatic balance even in well-trained, healthy men (Table 1). These unfavorable changes were, however, more evident in men with a higher level of coronary risk factors such as hypercholesterolemia and mild hypertension and in men over 50 years of age. In the post-infarction patients we have observed much higher activation of blood platelets and a diminished

Table 1   Schematic Representation of Exercise-Induced Haemostatic Changes in Healthy Adult Men Based on Authors' Own Experimental Studies Performed 1983-1986.

Exercise	Platelet activation	Coagulation activation	Antithrombin III activity	Fibrinolytic activity	Haemostatic activity
Moderate, short-term isometric exercise	0	0	−	0	0
Moderate, 20-min aerobic, endurance exercise	0	0 or +	0 or +	+	0
Moderate, prolonged (60 min), aerobic exercise	0	0 or +	+ or 0	+ or + +	0
Maximum, short-term, anaerobic exercise	+ or + +	+	+ or 0	+ +	unfavorable changes in some subjects
Strenuous, prolonged exercise (marathon race)	+ or + +	+ or + +	+	+ +	unfavorable changes in some subjects

Note. + rise; 0 unchanged; − unknown.

response of fibrinolysis due to anaerobic exercise as compared with healthy controls. Moderate 20-min aerobic exercise led to a marked increase of fibrinolytic activity without any considerable activation of blood platelet and coagulation both in CHD patients and in healthy untrained individuals. The experiments have demonstrated that the time interval between successive bouts of prolonged exercise may significantly influence the haemostatic response.

In order to take advantage of all the benefits of regular exercise as well as to reduce the frequency of cardiac fatalities it seems necessary to elaborate the new physiopathological approach toward the preventive and rehabilitative training programs with regard to the exercise-induced haemostatic changes. It seems that analysis of exercise-induced haemostatic changes may increase the possibility of identifying and warning individuals who are at special risk of myocardial infarction or sudden death during exercise, and should allow the creation of less harmful training programs as a contribution to CHD prevention and rehabilitation.

References

Drygas, W.K., Röcker, L., Boldt, F., Heyduck, B., & Altenkirch, H.U. (1986). *Der Einfluss einer standardisierten aeroben und anaeroben ergometrischen Belastung auf das Hämostase und Fibrinolysesystem bei Gesunden und Herzinfarktpatienten.* Deutscher Sportärztekongress, Kiel (abstr. 42).

Drygas, W.K. (in press). Changes in blood platelet function and fibrinolytic activity in response to moderate, exhaustive and prolonged exercise in normal men. *Int. J. Sports Med.*

Jokl, E. (1975). Syncope in athletes. *Five monographs*, 71-269.

Röcker, L., Stiege-Quast, B., Schwandt, H.J., & Quast, J. (1984). Der Einfluss körperlicher Leistung auf die Antithrombin-III-Aktivität im Plasma. In D. Jeschke (Ed.), *Position of sports medicine in medicine and sports science*. Springer Verlag, Berlin, 482-485.

Röcker, L., Drygas, W.K., & Heyduck, B. (1986). Blood platelet activation and increase in thrombin activity following a marathon race. *Eur. J. Appl. Physiol.*, **55**, 374-380.

Samek, L., Ritter, B., Schöll, B.V., Gohlke, H., Betz, P., Weidemann, H., Schnellbacher, K., & Roskamm, H. (1982). Herzinfarkt während sportlicher Aktivität. In *Sport Leistung und Gesundheit*. Kongressbd. Dtsch. Sportärztekongress.

Shephard, R.J. (1984). Applications of exercise and training in coronary heart disease. *Int. J. Sports Med.*, **5**, 49-53.

Wybitul, K., Thiel, M., Keller, E., Lindenmaier, M., & Merten R. (1983). Der plötzliche Tod beim. *Sport. Med. Welt*, **34**, 1098-1102.

The Effect of Increased Physical Activity for 3 to 4 Years After Myocardial Infarction on the Course of Coronary Heart Disease: A 12-Year Follow-Up Study

L. Ziółkowski

Department of Applied Physiology, Medical Research Centre, Polish Academy of Sciences, Warsaw, Poland

Beneficial effects of increased physical activity in coronary patients after myocardial infarction (MI) have not been explicitly proved, although it is often recommended to the patients (Denolin, 1980; Kallio, 1983; Naughton, 1976). Thus, the purpose of this work was to evaluate an influence of increased physical activity for 3 to 4 years on work tolerance and responses of the cardiovascular system to exercise tests examined immediately after completing the training program, and then a few years following termination of the training. This work makes a part of the longitudinal (12 years) follow-up study of coronary heart disease (CHD) after the first myocardial infarction.

Material and Methods

One hundred forty-one male patients, after the first uncomplicated myocardial infarction (MI) were included in this study. All of them were "white-collar workers," fit to perform physical exercise. They were divided into 2 groups: patients of group A ($n = 63$, age 64.8 ± 6.2 years) participated in the low-intensity training program for 3 to 4 years, whereas patients of group B ($n = 78$, age 48 ± 7.2 years), who maintained their most sedentary daily routine, served as controls.

The weekly training program of group A consisted of 8 to 10 h of self-controlled walking at the speed of 4 to 6 km $\cdot$ h^{-1}, 2 h of supervised walking + calisthenics. The speed of walking was predetermined based on the energy cost $\dot{V}O_2$ and heart rate (HR) during the ergometer exercise test (Kallio, 1983; Kozłowski, Nazar, & Chwalbińska-Moneta, 1984; Kozłowski, Ziółkowski, & Nazar, 1984; Ziółkowski, 1986). The first training program sessions had begun a few months after MI, following the hospital and sanatorium treatment.

The cycloergometer exercise test (ET) with the work load increasing from 50 W by 12.5 W every 6 min was continued until appearance of significant ECG changes (e.g., ST depression > 2 mm, arrhythmias, or when the patients reached the submaximal work load of 60-70% HR$_{max}$. During the exercise test oxygen uptake ($\dot{V}O_2$), cardiac output ($\dot{Q}$), by CO_2 rebreathing method, and blood lactate (LA) concentration were measured. Based on these measurements the relative work load (% HR$_{max}$), $\dot{V}O_2$max, and the ratios between $\dot{Q}$ and $\dot{V}O_2$ were calculated. The ST depression was related both to the absolute and relative work loads, using the following indices: ST depression $\times \dot{V}O_2^{-1}$ and ST depression $\times$ % HR$_{max}^{-1}$, respectively (Ziółkowski, 1986).

At the end of the 12-year follow up period the following groups of patients were distinguished:

1. Patients with slight deterioration of clinical state but without any severe complications (37 patients from group A, 33 patients from group B);

2. Patients with marked deterioration, with complications such as cardiac insufficiency, arrhythmia, etc. (10 patients from group A, 17 patients from group B); and

3. Patients who deceased during 12 years (18 patients from group A, 26 patients from group B).

Results

Three years after MI, working capacity of the patients from group A was markedly higher than that of the patients from group B. The tolerance of work load ($\dot{V}O_2$) during ET was greater in the trained patients and their cardiac output ($\dot{Q}$) was much higher with a similar heart rate ($p < .05$). The ST-segment depression in ECG was smaller in group A. Seven years after MI (i.e., 3-4 years following termination of the training program), differences between the groups were markedly diminished. Although the patients from group A still tolerated greater exercise loads and attained higher $\dot{Q}$ values during the test, the magnitude of their ST depression in ECG was similar to that in the patients from group B. An analysis of the 12-year course of coronary heart disease after MI revealed that patients from group A and B did not differ significantly in the incidence of cardiac deaths (group III) or severe aggravation of the disease (group II).

Conclusions

1. The above presented program of increasing physical activity for patients after myocardial infarction was well tolerated by all the patients in spite of differences in their working capacity and a degree of coronary insufficiency.

2. The training program applied for a period of 3 to 4 years after MI, consisting of physical exercise of low or moderate intensities (30-50% HR_{max}) performed 8 to 12 h per week, resulted in significant improvement of the patients' work tolerance.

3. After 3 years of the training the cardiovascular response to physical exercise was also improved. The patients who participated in this program (group A) reached greater cardiac output ($\dot{Q}$) and attained lower blood LA concentration in response to a given work load than the patients leading sedentary life (group B).

4. Seven years after MI (i.e., 3-4 years after cessation of the supervised training), the differences between groups were markedly diminished, and all the patients showed a similar degree of ischemia as reflected by ST depression in the exercise ECG.

5. An analysis of the 12-year course of CHD after MI failed to reveal any differences between physically active and sedentary patients in the incidence of cardiac death or severe aggravation of the disease.

Acknowledgments

This work was supported by the Polish Central Programme of Basic Research 06-02-III.1.9.

References

Cobb, F.R., Williams, R.S., McEwan, P., Jones, R.H., Coleman, R.E., & Wallace, A.G. (1982). Effects of exercise training on ventricular function in patients with recent myocardial infarction. *Circulation,* **66**, 100-108.

Denolin, H. (1980). L'activité physique a-t-elle un effet préventif dans le développment de la maladie coronaire? *Kard. Pol.,* **23**, 913-915.

Kallio, V. (1983). The influence of physical rehabilitation and risk-factor control on long-term prognosis of postinfarction patients. In H. Roskamm (Ed.), *Prognosis of coronary heart disease progression of coronary arteriosclerosis.* Springer-Verlag, Berlin, 196-206.

Kozłowski, S., Nazar, K., & Chwalbińska-Moneta, J. (1984). Role of physical activity in clinical medicine. In S. Kozłowski and K. Nazar (Eds.), *Introduction to clinical physiology.* PZWL, Warsaw, 345-355.

Kozłowski, S., Ziółkowski, L., & Nazar, K. (1984). Physical exercise and internal diseases. In S. Kozłowski and K. Nazar (Eds.), *Introduction to clinical physiology.* PZWL, Warsaw, 378-423.

Naughton, J. (1976). Rehabilitation after myocardial infarction. In J.I. Haft & Ch.P. Bailey (Eds.), *Advances in the management of clinical heart disease.* Future Publ. Comp., New York.

Zohman, L.R., Young, J.L., & Kattus, A.A. (1983). Treadmill walking protocol for the diagnostic evaluation and exercise programming of cardiac patients. *Am. J. Cardiol.,* **51**, 1081-1086.

Ziółkowski, L. (1986). Indices of coronary insufficiency in exercise ecg: 12 year-longitudinal study in patients after myocardial infarction. *Bull. Pol. Acad. Sci.,* **34**, 173-185.

Long-Term Physical Training and Cardiovascular Function, Lipid Metabolism, and the Blood Clotting System in Men After Acute Myocardial Infarction

K. Moczurad and A.M. Curyło

Department of Social Cardiology and I Department of Cardiology, Institute of Cardiology, Academy of Medicine, Kraków, Poland

Physical training in patients after myocardial infarction (MI) has been objectively recognized as a significant factor modifying survival, reinfarction rate, and certain coronary risk factors. However, most studies have dealt with these effects separately. Therefore, we have decided to examine certain factors that might play a role in further development of the disease and to evaluate modifying effects of graded physical training.

Material and Methods

A group of 202 men aged 30 to 64 years (mean age = 50.8), after the first MI, was followed for 5 years. We studied the effects of physical training on the cardiovascular system by using multigraded bicycle stress testing, electrocardiographic recordings, and left ventricular systolic time intervals (STI) measuring. The influence of long-term physical training on the blood clotting system and serum lipoproteins was also investigated. The evaluations were repeated every 3 months for 5 years. Group I consisted of 86 patients undergoing interval supervised training, group II of 56 patients undergoing nonsupervised training and group III, 60 control patients.

Results

Over 5 years there were 3 deaths (3.5%) in group I, 5 (8.9%) in group II, and 6 (10.0%) in group III. Reinfarctions occurred in all groups, but they were most frequent in the control group; in group I, 3 patients (3.5%), group II, 5 patients (8.9%), and group III, 11 patients (18.3%). These differences were found significant ($p < .01$). We observed also significant differences between the groups in the incidence of anginal pain, rhythm disturbances, and exercise-induced ST-T segment changes in the ECG. They occurred in 8 patients (9.6%) of group I, 9 patients (17.6%) of group II, and 16 patients (29.6%) of group III. The numbers of rehospitalized patients over the 5-year-studies were as follows: in group I, 6 patients (6.9%); in group II, 6 (10.7%); and in group III, 19 patients (31.6%).

Results of determining the left ventricular systolic time intervals are not unequivocal, but we could detect shortening of the left ventricular ejection time index (LVETI) after exercise testing in group I. This tendency could not be found in groups II and III. Similarly the ratio of the preejection period (PEP) to left ventricular ejection time (LVET), thought to be a valuable indicator of contractility, showed the greatest decreasing tendency in the supervised training group (Levis et al., 1977).

Laboratory studies in group I in the first year of rehabilitation revealed a consistent decrease in blood triglyceride, pre-beta-lipoprotein and beta-lipoprotein levels with a simultaneous increase in alpha-lipoprotein and alpha-cholesterol levels. In the second year of rehabilitation alpha-cholesterol and alpha-lipoprotein increased further, reaching the level of significance ($p < .001$) after 86 weeks (Table 1). Neither in groups II nor III were any significant changes in the measured variables observed. The studies of the blood clotting system showed that bleeding time and euglobulin lysis time were significantly prolonged, primarily in group I (Table 1).

Discussion

The results of the studies showed an importance of physical training as a mode of rehabilitation after MI, although its role in coronary heart disease has been recently questioned (Ellestad, 1987). Suitable interval physical training significantly affected the cardiovascular system in patients after MI, resulting both in a significant decrease in the reinfarction rate and in the sudden death rate. In contrast, the results of eight controlled prevention trials, using physical training after MI, have not shown any significant decrease in the mortality and reinfarction rates (Naughton, 1983). However, seven of them have revealed that mortality tended to decrease in the training groups.

Physical training may have beneficial effects on several atherosclerosis risk factors (Dufaux et al., 1982; Wood & Haskell, 1979). Our studies showed its favorable influence on the serum lipoprotein level that occurred in the first year of rehabilitation and enhanced in the second year. Changes in the blood clotting system (i.e., prolongation of bleeding time and euglobulin lysis time) as well as the results of STI are rather controversial (Weiss, 1980). The exercise-induced shortening of LVETI and a decrease in the PEP/LVET ratio is interpreted by some authors as the result of improvement of left ventricular contractility (Whitsett & Naughton, 1971).

Conclusions

1. Supervised interval training of patients during 5 years after MI produces a significant decrease in the incidence of reinfarctions and a fall in sudden cardiac deaths as well as in rhythm disturbances, anginal attacks, and ST-T segment changes in the exercise ECG.

2. In training patients the left ventricular performance improves, which manifests itself in the shortening of LVETI and a decrease in the PEP/LVET ratio.

3. Patients of the supervised training group exhibited a significant decrease in blood lipid fractions known as atherogenic with simultaneous increase in fractions protecting against atherosclerosis.

4. These findings indicate an important role of an organized form of physical training for patients after myocardial infarction.

References

Dufaux, B., Assman, G., & Hollmann, W. (1982). Plasma lipoproteins and physical activity: A review. *Int. J. Sports Med., 3*, 123-136.

Ellestad, M.H. (1987). Is exercise harmful in ischemic heart disease? *Am. J. Noninvas. Cardiol., 1*, 15-17.

Table 1   Selected Parameters of Blood Clotting System and Plasma Lipoproteins in Group I of Supervised Training

	Before training	After 1 yr	After 2 yr	After 3 yr	After 4 yr	After 5 yr
Bleeding time (sec)	211. ± 47.2 NS	261. ± 68.4[a]	288. ± 69.8[c]	286. ± 70.1[a]	279. ± 68.0[a]	281. ± 64.0[a]
Euglobulin lysis time (min)	152. ± 11.2 NS	165. ± 18.1 NS	173. ± 12.2[c]	174. ± 16.2[a]	172. ± 18.0[a]	175. ± 18.8[a]
Alpha-lipoproteins (%)	21.9 ± 6.3 NS	25.1 ± 5.1[a]	26.5 ± 4.2[d]	25.4 ± 5.4[a]	25.8 ± 5.0[b]	25.6 ± 5.3[a]
Alpha-cholesterol (mmol/L)	1.10 ± 0.21 NS	1.18 ± 0.19[b]	1.19 ± 0.21[a]	1.15 ± 0.22 NS	1.14 ± 0.20 NS	1.13 ± 0.19 NS

Note. NS = not significant. [a] $p = .05$, [b] $p = .02$, [c] $p = .01$, [d] $p = .001$.

Levis, R.P., Rittgers, S.E., Forester, W.F., & Boudoulas, H. (1977). A critical review of the systolic time intervals. *Circulation, 56*, 146-158.

Naughton, J. (1983). Death rates of cardiac patients: Effects of physical activity. *Prim. Cardiol., 9*, 77-85.

Weiss, H.J. (1980). Platelets and ischemic heart disease. *N. Engl. J. Med., 302*, 225-229.

Whitsett, T.L., & Naughton, R.T. (1971). Effect of exercise on systolic time intervals in sedentary and active individuals and rehabilitated patients with heart disease. *Am. J. Cardiol., 27*, 352-361.

Wood, P.D., & Haskell, W.L. (1979). The effect of exercise on plasma high density lipoproteins. *Lipids, 14*, 417-427.

Application of the Ergometric Test With a Static Load Component in the Diagnosis and Evaluation of Coronary Insufficiency

E. Wójcik-Ziółkowska

Department of Applied Physiology, Medical Research Centre, Polish Academy of Sciences, Warsaw, Poland

The main goal in constant searching for exercise tests of high diagnostic value is an increase in their sensitivity, ensuring the earliest precise detection of coronary insufficiency (Kerber et al., 1975). It has been proved that static exercises considerably increase cardiac oxygen demand (Katori et al., 1976; Kilbom & Persson, 1981; Kozłowski & Nazar, 1984; Lowe et al., 1975; Perez et al., 1980). Thus, the aim of this work was to elucidate usefulness of the dynamic exercise test with a static load component in an early diagnosis and evaluation of the degree of coronary insufficiency.

Material and Methods

Two groups of patients were examined: group I (RF), consisting of 26 asymptomatic subjects (mean age 48.0 $\pm$ 8.3 years) with coronary heart disease (CHD) risk factors (e.g., hyperlipidemia, unstable hypertension, obesity), and group II (CHD), consisting of 25 patients (mean age 55.1 $\pm$ 5.2 years) with clinically diagnosed CHD, in majority after the first uncomplicated myocardial infarction.

The study was performed in 2 stages. In the first stage patients of both groups performed the mixed exercise test (MT). For this purpose the standard ergometer test was modified in such a way that during the dynamic work with increasing intensity the patients were holding in one hand 2 to 4 kg of weight fixed to the cycloergometer handle, using the block mechanical system. Duration of the test was limited by appearance of ischemia symptoms in the exercise ECG or subjective symptoms, mainly upper extremity pain caused by holding the weight. In the second stage, a standard ergometric test (ET) was performed. The sequence and magnitude of dynamic exercise loads as well as the duration of the test were the same as in MT.

During both exercise tests ECG was continuously monitored from 4 chest electrodes, and heart rate (HR) was calculated. Blood pressure (BP) was measured every 1 min. Oxygen uptake ($\dot{V}O_2$) and cardiac output ($\dot{Q}$—CO_2 rebreathing method) were measured in the last minute of the tests.

Results

It was found that the static component added to the dynamic load in the standard cyclo-ergometer test did not increase its energy cost. In spite of that, the heart work, as expressed by the double product $DP = BP_s \times HR \times 10^{-2}$, was significantly higher in MT than in

ET because of the markedly enhanced BP response to the former test. The cardiac output ($\dot{Q}$) during MT attained lower values in comparison with ET because of lower stroke volume. In both groups of patients (RF and CHD) more pronounced ischemic changes in the exercise ECG were found in MT in comparison with ET. Thus, the static load added to the dynamic work allowed to reveal ischemic changes in the exercise ECG in many subjects previously considered as asymptomatic. In addition, MT disclosed the ventricular rhythm disturbances in some patients from groups I and II. In conclusion, this study revealed usefulness of the applied mixed test in diagnosis of coronary insufficiency in patients considered as asymptomatic based on a standard diagnostic exercise procedure.

Acknowledgments

This work was supported by the Polish Central Programme of Basic Research 06-02-III.1.9.

References

Katori, R., Miyzawa, K., Ikeda, S., Shirato, K., Muraguchi, I., & Hayashi, T. (1976). Coronary blood flow and lactate metabolism isometric handgrip exercise in heart disease. *Jap. Heart J.*, **17**, 742.

Kerber, R.E., Miller, R.A., & Najjar, S.M. (1975). Myocardial ischemic effects of isometric, dynamic and combined exercise in coronary artery disease. *Chest*, **67**, 388.

Kilbom, A., & Persson, J. (1981). Cardiovascular response to combined dynamic and static exercise. *Circ. Res.*, **1**(Suppl. I), 48.

Kozłowski, S., & Nazar, K. (1984). Static exercise. In S. Kozłowski and K. Nazar (Eds.), *Introduction to clinical physiology*. PZWL, Warsaw, 276-281.

Lowe, D.K., Rothbaum, D.A., McHenry, O.L., Corya, B.C., & Knoebel, S.B. (1975). Myocardial blood flow response to isometric (handgrip) and treadmill exercise in coronary artery disease. *Circulation*, **51**, 26.

Perez, J.E., Cintron, G., Gonzales, M., Hernandez, E., Linares, E., & Aranda, J.M. (1980). Hemodynamic response to isometric handgrip in acute myocardial infarction. *Chest*, **77**, 194.

Long-Term Benefits of Regular Exercise in Coronary Heart Disease Prevention: The Problem of Threshold Dose of Physical Activity

W. Drygas, H. Kuński, and A. Jegier

Department of Sports Medicine, Medical Academy, Łódź, Poland

It is generally accepted that individuals of all ages should be encouraged to develop a physically active lifestyle as part of a comprehensive program for disease prevention and health promotion. However, most data concerning beneficial effects of physical training are based on cross-sectional or short-term experimental studies. Only a few data are available concerning prolonged effects of regular exercise. Therefore, the purpose of our study was a long-term prospective observation of systematical training in middle-aged men. In this paper we present preliminary data of a 5-year continuous (year-by-year) and 5-year follow-up study in the group of asymptomatic men aged 30 to 59 (mean 44.2) involved in regular endurance training (running, jogging, tennis, swimming) for several years (mean 6.5 years).

The data from the 5-year follow-up study in 25 men who had trained about 4.8 h weekly have demonstrated that further regular training led to a significant improvement in aerobic capacity (PWC 150 increased by 28% from 174 to 223 W, $p < .001$) and marked changes in systolic (128 vs 120, $p < .02$) and diastolic blood pressure (92 vs 81, $p < .001$). Body weight (74.8 vs 75.2 kg), body fat (15.0 vs 15.6%), and LBM (63.5 vs 63.4 kg) did not change significantly during exercise. Some positive but statistically insignificant alterations in cholesterol (5.76 vs 5.49 mmol/L) and HDL cholesterol concentration (1.27 vs 1.30 mmol/L) were noted. However, the ratio chol:HDL decreased significantly from 4.54 to 4.22; $p < .02$. Due to the changes in several coronary risk factors, the total coronary risk ratio decreased markedly by 22.2% from 9.0 to 7.0; $p < .01$. Similar trends have been observed in year-by-year observation in 22 men.

The extensive epidemiological study (Polish Trial on Coronary Heart Disease Prevention) performed in the comparable time has demonstrated an increase in several coronary risk factors and total coronary risk in the general population of Poland. The data from our 5-year prospective observation strongly suggest that in well motivated middle-aged men involved for several years in endurance training, further positive modification of coronary risk factors is possible, provided that the threshold dose of physical activity is exceeded. In order to define the minimum dose of exercise effective for health promotion and modification of selected coronary risk factors, we carried out a cross-sectional study in 146 men and a long-term prospective observation (mean 3.7 years) in 69 men with different levels of leisure time physical activity. These data have demonstrated that energy expenditure of 1000-1499 kcal/week due to moderate, regular endurance training with intensity of 5 kcal/min is sufficient to improve aerobic capacity and to modify beneficially several coronary risk factors. Assuming that modification of selected risk factors may reduce the frequency of CHD, one may suppose that regular, moderate endurance training connected with energy expenditure above 1000 kcal/week may be an important factor in primary prevention of coronary heart disease.

The Effect of Sanatorium Rehabilitation on the Psychophysiological State of Patients After Myocardial Infarction

S. Rudnicki, J. Tylka, Z. Kobak, and I. Kubacka

Clinic and Department of Cardiac Rehabilitation, National Institute of Cardiology, Warsaw, Poland

The aim of this study was to evaluate psychophysiological states and vocational activities of patients who had MI approximately 10 years ago. Moreover, an attempt was made to evaluate advantages of the 28-day sanatorium rehabilitation organized for these patients. Forty-eight male individuals under 60 years of age were randomly selected from the population of MI patients undergoing the posthospital rehabilitation in 1975 and 1976. Before MI, 47 (99.9%) patients were occupationally active. During the 12 months after completion of the posthospital rehabilitation 45 (93.7%) patients returned to their jobs. Ten years later 33 persons (70%) were still working. The average work time was shortened after MI from 12.3 to 7 hours per day. Twenty-four patients (50%) remained at the full-time work schedule and 9 (18%) were employed part-time. Prior to the admittance to the sanatorium all patients were subjected to the submaximal exercise test; 42% of them had a relatively good work tolerance and they were in a steady period of the coronary heart disease. Four patients (8.3%) were excluded from the physical rehabilitation program because of contraindications for any kind of exercise.

The psychological testing of patients showed that they had a sense of inferiority, subordinance, and extravertic desire to be helped. A comparison of the real and ideal self-image indicated a relatively low level of patients' self-approval. Twenty patients were classified as "A" type of behavior while 28 presented the "B" type. In the initial stage of the study 80% of the type "A" and 61% of the type "B" patients manifested a relatively high anxiety level. In both groups a statistically significant decrease of the anxiety tension, along with an increase in the positive attitude towards the therapy was observed during the 4-week period of rehabilitation. Thus, the study revealed that the resumption of the rehabilitation treatment was positively reflected in the emotional sphere of the patients.

Part VII
Research Abstracts

Changes in Physical Working Capacity During the Second Decade of Life: A Longitudinal Study

B. Woynarowska

Department of School Medicine, National Research Institute of Mother and Child, Warsaw, Poland

Serial data were analyzed for PWC_{170} recorded semiannually between the ages of 12 and 19 years for 64 boys and girls. There were two groups: sports group (S, $n = 20$) for children participating in sports at school or clubs, and nonsports group (NS, $n = 44$). PWC_{170} was calculated from measurements of heart rate and work load during three submaximal exercises on a bicycle ergometer (Monark). The mean values of PWC_{170} were higher in S groups than in NS groups at the initial measurements and the differences between these groups increased with age and became significant especially in boys. In boys 6% of the variance of PWC_{170} changes were accounted for by participation in sports and 53% by age. The corresponding percentages of variance for girls were 12% and 24%, respectively.

There was a tendency to level off the PWC_{170} values at the period one year before and after menarche in girls in group S and NS. In boys mean values of PWC_{170} increased systematically during puberty and the increments were the highest 0.5 to 1 year after the peak height velocity. The correlation coefficients between the levels of PWC_{170} at age 12 and 19 years were in girls, group S, $r = .78$ and group NS, $r = .19$; in boys 0.37 and 0.49, respectively. Because of the large S_{EE} the error of PWC_{170} estimation at the age of 19 years from the value at age 12 years was 15% in boys and 20% in girls.

Aerobic and Anaerobic Energy Production in Speed Skiing

E. Rauhala, J. Karvonen, and Y. Kumpula

Department of Physiology, University of Kuopio, Finland

The aim of this study was to find out the role of aerobic and anaerobic energy production in speed skiing. Subjects were five 20 to 30-year-old representatives of the Finnish Speed Skiing Association. The subjects did three consecutive speed runs on a 750-m long course with a height difference of 171 m and an average slope of 45%. Running speeds were measured, as well as capillary blood lactic acid concentrations three minutes after the end of, and heart rates during, each run. In the second run, running speed was 135.65 ± 3.88 km $\cdot$ h^{-1} and in the third run 137.63 ± 5.41 km $\cdot$ h^{-1} ($p > .05$). Capillary blood lactic acid concentration after the first run was 3.20 ± 1.39 mmol $\cdot$ L^{-1} and after the third run 2.80 ± 0.94 mmol $\cdot$ L^{-1} ($p > .05$). Maximal heart rate during the first run was 169 ± 8 min^{-1} and during the third run 163 ± 3 min^{-1} ($p > .05$). Speed skiing imposed a maximal load neither on the anaerobic nor on the aerobic capacity. It can be concluded that performance in speed skiing depends on the alactic anaerobic capacity (ATP, creatine phosphate), the degree of relaxation, neuromuscular coordination, muscular strength, and factors decreasing air resistance.

Physiological Characteristics of Fencing

B. Psyta and H.D. Halicka-Ambroziak

Department of Physiology, Academy of Physical Education, Warsaw, Poland

The aim of this study was to evaluate physiological reactions during specific exercise in fencing. Six representatives of Academic Club (range 18-23 years) participated in the study. Maximal aerobic power was assessed by using a progressive test conducted on a cycle ergometer. Subjects had a mean $\pm$ SD VO_2max 3.56 $\pm$ 0.41 L $\cdot$ min^{-1} (49.87 $\pm$ 7.24 ml $\cdot$ min^{-1} $\cdot$ kg^{-1}). Three pairs of fencers were fighting three times (5 min each time) with a 5-min break between every fight. Oxygen consumption was measured continuously during specific work and recovery. Heart rate was registered telemetrically (Medinik). During rest and 2 min after finishing the exercise capillary blood lactate was estimated. Mean $\pm$ SD oxygen consumption during the fight was 2.31 $\pm$ 0.38 L $\cdot$ min^{-1}. The range of heart rate during fencing was 117 to 170 beats $\cdot$ min^{-1}. The heart rate during the last minute of exercise was 149 $\pm$ 14 beats $\cdot$ min^{-1}. Blood lactate 2 min after exercise was 2.00 $\pm$ 0.12 mmol $\cdot$ L^{-1}.

Biofeedback Technique in Evaluating Pilots' Performance Capacity

S. Barański, F. Skibniewski, F. Klukowski, and J. Olton
Military Institute of Aviation Medicine, Warsaw, Poland

Up to now many noninvasive tests of the circulatory system function, including evaluation of hypoxia effects, have been used in pilots. However, there is no routine protocol of tests evaluating hypoxia tolerance in pilots under different exercise loads. In this study an attempt was made to develop an applicable program for the above mentioned tests.

To fulfill this purpose the following prerequisites were considered: (a) repeated increasing submaximal workloads should not exceed 70 to 75% of the maximal heart rate (HR_{max}); (b) the work time should be approximately 10 min; and (c) the applied workloads should allow the subjects, who are unadapted to altitude, to work in moderate hypoxia. In the exercise test the biofeedback method (HR-workload) was applied. Based on the assigned levels of the steady state HR, changes in power output and total work done provide indices for the subjects' physical capacity.

The study included 11 healthy fit men, aged 23.4 ± 2.1 years, body weight 68.8 ± 10.2 kg, height 176.6 ± 6.9 cm. The Fizjotest-801 made by Medipan (Poland) was applied to control the Elema-Schönander bicycle ergometer workloads. Heart rate and power output were monitored and ecg was recorded. The exercise test was performed twice. On the first day it was carried out under normobaric conditions in a low pressure chamber (LPCh). On the second day the subjects performed the exercise test at simulated altitude of 3000 m a.s.l. (LPCh), after a 20-min rest at that altitude. The test consisted of the following stages: 1-min initial data registration; 3-min warming up at HR_{100}; three 3-min workload bouts at HR_{145}, HR_{150}, HR_{145} preceded by 1-min, 1-min, and 2-min intervals, respectively.

In the exercise test the following indices were analyzed: P_m—mean power output (W) in each min of the 3-min bout; P_p—peak power output (W) during the linearly increasing phase of exercise; L—total mechanical work (kJ and J · kg^{-1}); t_a—time needed to attain the peak power (s). For comparison of mean differences the student t test for paired variables was applied.

The obtained results showed that under moderate hypoxia (3000 m a.s.l.) the mean and peak power outputs were significantly lower ($p < .01$) at the steady state HR values in comparison with those under standard conditions (P_p decreased from 227.8 ± 45.6 to 209 ± 41.0 W; P_m, from 185.8 ± 37.5 to 164.5 ± 35.6 W). Decreases in the mechanical parameters were from 3 to 8%. The t_a proved to be of the least prognostic value. The total mechanical work decreased under hypoxic conditions by 12% from 139.0 ± 24.1 to 122.1 ± 18.0 J · kg^{-1} ($p < .01$).

Conclusions

1. The presented 3-bout repeated submaximal exercise test (with biofeedback HR-workload monitoring) allows an estimation of working capacity in healthy men under conditions of moderate altitude hypoxia.

2. A significant decrease (by 12%) in the total mechanical work was demonstrated under altitude hypoxia, as compared to the standard conditions. Other indices decreased from 3% to 8%.

3. The dynamics of the heart rate recovery were similar at standard conditions, and at 3000 m a.s.l. in spite of the difference in the total work output.

Discriminative Reaction Time During Graded Exercise in Girls Aged 16 to 19 Years

J. Chmura

Department of Physiology, Academy of Physical Education in Wrocław and the District Sports Medicine Unit in Jelenia Góra, Poland

This study was performed with 46 girls aged 16.3 $\pm$ 0.5 years whose mean $\dot{V}O_2$max was 2.64 $\pm$ 0.28 L $\cdot$ m^{-1} (group 1) and 30 girls aged 18.2 $\pm$ 0.8 years whose $\dot{V}O_2$max was 3.32 $\pm$ 0.31 L $\cdot$ min^{-1} (group 2). They were subjected to the discriminative audio-visual tests before, during, and after graded bicycle ergometer exercise. The work intensity was increased by 50 W every 6 min, starting from 50 W to a maximal load. The reaction time was measured during the last 2 min of each exercise load and then every 5 min of the recovery period. Heart rate and oxygen uptake were recorded continuously.

At rest the mean reaction time was significantly shorter in group 2 (0.402 s) than in group 1 (0.425 s) and in both the groups it decreased with increment of work load up to approximately 70 to 75% $\dot{V}O_2$max (0.366 and 0.396 s, respectively), increasing above these values in the final period of exercise (0.382 and 0.414 s, respectively). However, in 11 girls of group 1 and 12 from group 2 a progressive decrease in the reaction time up to the maximal load was noted. These subgroups (1A and 2A) showed better psychomotor responsiveness and had higher work capacity in comparison with the remaining age-matched girls. In all girls examined, further reduction in the reaction time was found during the recovery period with the lowest values at 10 to 11 min in group 1 (0.393 s) and at 15 to 16 min in group 2 (0.359 s). In both groups the number of correct responses was increased both during and after exercise as compared to the pre-exercise score.

The data demonstrated that physical exercise causes an improvement of psychomotor responsiveness. In a majority of cases the shortest reaction time during exercise occurs at 70 to 75% $\dot{V}O_2$max, although in approximately 30% of the girls examined the best results were achieved at the higher work intensities. Further shortening of the reaction time occurs within 15 min of the recovery period. The study indicates that testing of psychomotor ability during and after exercise could be useful in evaluating the tolerance of physical fatigue in athletes.

Immunological Response to Physical Effort

B. Wit

Institute of Biological Sciences, Department of Physiology, Warsaw, Poland

Many authors have reported a high incidence of infections in athletes undergoing intensive training, preceding the starting period. In the present study the following problems were examined: to what extent regular training affects the responses of immunological resistance measured at a cell level; whether the training load applied to athletes disturbs their humoral resistance; and whether the level of immunoglobulins changes during the training cycle in systematically training athletes.

This study included 217 athletes of four sport disciplines and four control groups. In distance runners, cell resistance tests and humoral resistance tests were performed (lymphocyte transformation test—LTT, migration inhibition test—MIT, T, and B lymphocyte counts, as well as concentrations of immunoglobulins IgG, IgA, and IgM). In gymnasts, canoeists, and swimmers the immunoglobulin level (IgG, IgA, IgM) was determined on NOR-Partigen plates. In gymnasts, measurements were repeated three times with 12-month intervals, whereas in canoeists and swimmers they were performed during various periods of the training cycle. Similar measurements were also made in the control groups. More pronounced changes occurred in the humoral resistance parameters as compared to those in the cell resistance indicators. A decrease in the immunoglobulin level to the lower limits of physiological values was noted at the period of competitions and just prior to it. One should also note the nonspecific activation of the immunological system during the intermediate periods of the training cycle.

Knee Extension and Flexion and EMG Level in Different Angles of Flexion

T. Sihvonen, J. Honkanen, O. Airaksinen, K. Baskin, and O. Hänninen

Department of Physiology, University of Kuopio and University Central Hospital of Kuopio, Finland

Patellar stability in lateral direction is very important to normal patellofemoral function. Possible imbalance of activity between vastus lateralis and vastus medialis muscles can be seen especially in the late extension. The most effective way to activate the patellar extensor system has been subject to discussion. In this study we measured the maximal isometric extension and flexion forces of the right knee in eight ice hockey players with Cybex Orthotrom isokinetic equipment. The knee was adjusted to 5, 30, 60, and 90 degrees flexion. At the same time, we also measured EMG activity from the motor point with surface electrodes on v. medialis, v. lateralis, r. femoris, semitendinosus, and biceps femoris muscles. The total extension force was greatest at 60 degrees flexion (282 psi $\pm$ *SD* 61), and the correlation between total extension force and EMG activity of each entensor muscle was highest at this angle of flexion.

However, the greatest EMG activity level (1.2 mV $\pm$ *SD* 0.4) was measured at 90 degrees flexion. During flexion the EMG activity of flexor muscles was about the same between 5 and 60 degrees flexion and a significant correlation with total flexion force was noted in semitendinosus muscle only. We conclude that knee extensor muscles can be activated effectively against resistance at 60 to 90 degrees flexion and flexor muscles at 5 to 60 degrees flexion. For sport participants suffering from patellofemoral joint disturbances, isometric extensor exercises are recommended with the knee at 60 to 90 degrees of flexion. Also the contact stress (Kg $\times$ cm) in the patellofemoral joint is lowest at this flexion angle.

The Effect of Prolonged Endurance Training on In Vitro Tissue Metabolism

R. Jusiak

Department of Physiology, Academy of Physical Education, Warsaw, Poland

The aim of this work was to evaluate metabolic changes in rat tissues during a long-term endurance training (group T) in comparison with untrained animals (group C). It was done by measuring oxygen uptake by tissue slices using the Warburg method. Half of the C and T animals were given vitamin B_{15} (Calgam) starting 12 days before their sacrifice. The treadmill training program included running 1 h per day for 5 days per week with increasing intensity up to 25 m $\cdot$ min^{-1} at 14% incline for 15 weeks. During 24 h preceding sacrifice the animals did not perform any forced activity, but were fed ad libitum the standard diet. Immediately after decapitation samples were taken from liver, myocardium, masseter m., soleus m., and the gastrocnemius types II-a and II-b muscle fibers both from C and T rats. Thin tissue slices were incubated for 1 h in the Warburg medium containing 0.15 M glucose.

The applied training caused a marked increase in O_2 uptake by slices of liver, myocardium, and the type II-a fibers of gastrocnemius, while in type II-b muscle fibers a decrease of O_2 uptake occurred. No such changes were found in soleus and masseter slices. Vitamin B_{15} administration decreased the uptake of O_2 by tissue slices from both C and T rats with an exception of slices from the fiber II-a of gastrocnemius m. The obtained results indicate that long-term endurance training results in enhanced increase in O_2 uptake by the liver, myocardium, and skeletal muscles consisting of fast twitching fibers. Vitamin B_{15} decreases tissue metabolism, at least in vitro.

Part VIII

Panel Discussion

Basic Physiological Factors Determining Endurance Performance

Bengt Saltin, Moderator

B. Saltin—There is a consensus that the heart capacity is most important for oxygen transport to working muscles. The intriguing problem concerns the cardiac enlargement induced by extremely intensive endurance training. The question arises, what is the factor limiting cardiac hypertrophy? Further, there are data suggesting that pericardium and not the cardiac muscle itself is responsible for this limitation. Another question is why the qualitative features of cardiac muscle are so difficult to change.

E. Jokl—Experiments with splitting the pericardium, carried out on greyhounds over 50 years ago, showed that these animals could perform better after the operation, thus suggesting that, indeed, as Prof. Saltin mentioned, the pericardium can limit physiological hypertrophy.

C. Jessen—I think that the fact that pathological enlargement of heart is more pronounced than the endurance training hypertrophy is not compatible with the hypothesis that pericardium limits the possibilities of physiological heart enlargement.

B. Saltin—This is an important point; and, we will have to explain in future studies whether the pericardium behaves differently under pathological and physiological conditions.

P.D. Gollnick—The heart may be considered as an almost self-trained organ, since daily human activities provide a constant stimulus sufficient to induce high oxygen capacity of cardiac muscle. Thus, physical training hardly evokes any further changes in the already high capacity of cardiac muscle to utilize oxygen.

There is a group of subjects who demonstrate a high increase in cardiac stroke volume—they are people fitted with fixed rate cardiac pacemakers. These people rely exclusively on the Frank–Starling mechanism for increasing their cardiac output. They can have extremely large stroke volumes, up to 200 ml. This indicates that the ability to increase cardiac stroke volume is fairly large, whereas the quality of heart muscle seems to be quite constant.

B. Saltin—Would you say that it is mainly an increase in venous return and then an enhancement in the right heart pressure that are responsible for the cardiac dilatation and hypertrophy?

P.D. Gollnick—Yes, that is probably true since the pressure in the pulmonary artery, which is normally somewhere around 7 to 12 mmHg in exercising normal subjects, and can go up to 15 to 20 mmHg in trained people, can reach 35 to 40 mmHg in patients with pacemakers. The fact that in normal people such a high pressure does not occur may be the reason for limitation in cardiac hypertrophy.

B. Saltin—The next problem to be discussed is to what extent distribution of cardiac output plays a role in limiting muscle perfusion. This problem seems to be particularly important in the light of the data obtained within the last five years demonstrating extremely high blood muscle perfusion values during exhausting exercise both in man and in some experimental animals.

R.L. Terjung—The local demands for blood flow are determined by the power output of the muscle. When a greater muscle mass is involved in exercise, there is a competition for cardiac output. The mechanism controlling the cardiac output distribution involves not only directing blood flow from the splanchnic area to muscles, but also from less to more engaged muscles. An issue that should be reconciled is how this is accomplished within the local and central regulatory systems.

B. Saltin—Under normal conditions, the central regulatory system is able to cope with the situation because blood pressure remains fairly constant. Where are sensors stimulating the sympathetic nervous system to constrict blood vessels to override locally elicited vasodilatator substances? Should one look for baroreceptors to be so sensitive that they can pick up beat-by-beat changes in peripheral conductance?

R.L. Terjung—Yes, it is possible. However, if an exercise becomes so strenuous that the resistance increases to high values a hypertensive response is observed. Now the afferent input from the periphery becomes more crucial and the experimental model with epidural anesthesia may prove beneficial in evaluating cardiovascular control.

C. Jessen—The mechanism regulating blood flow during exercise may be similar to that involved in thermoregulation. If an animal or human is exposed to a hot environment then peripheral vasodilation accompanied by splanchnic vasoconstriction occurs. This mechanism is triggered by the thermoreceptors themselves. There is an evidence for thermal afferents in skeletal muscles in goats. Both anatomists and histologists have described for many years some unmyelinated or sparsely myelinated nerve fibers in skeletal muscles with no specific functions attributed to them. One of the functions may be to transmit pain, another to signal the functional state of the muscle. They may sense, for example, pH, the level of potassium or temperature, and can be considered metabolic receptors. As such, they can trigger circulatory, respiratory, or thermoregulatory responses. It seems reasonable to have receptors close to the source of disturbance within the body. The mentioned nerve fibers can possibly be involved in setting limits to exercise.

E. Jokl—What is the physiological mechanism behind the enormous training-induced increase in strength and power output?

A. Bargossi—In my opinion, the increase in strength is in 80% due to the increase in muscle mass and in 20% to the central adaptation mechanisms. It is not clear to what extent the latter effect depends on changes in firing rate or motor unit recruitment.

P.D. Gollnick—Data from animals and human studies suggest that the tension produced per unit of a cross-sectional area of muscle is rather constant. So, we cannot look for any major changes with training in the force produced per unit of muscle. The only change we have seen in athletes for the last 20 years is an increase in muscle bulk. I know only one study in which muscle motor unit recruitment was compared before and after training (Milner-Brown, Stein, & Lee, 1975). The authors showed that in human muscles following training, there was more complete activation of the whole muscle. This is certainly an area worthy of further investigation.

B. Saltin—One of the topics that should be discussed is the mechanism of regulation of glycolysis, which is, of course, the main process yielding energy during a short-lasting event.

E. Hultman—Contraction and Ca^{2+} release are thought to be the most important regulators of glycolysis. We can get the maximum activation of phosphorylase with muscle stimulation within 1 to 2 s. Also an increase in inorganic phosphate (Pi) is important for regulation of glycolysis.

The last point we know very little about concerns the mechanism of reducing the rate of glycogenolysis with the time of exercise. If it is true that there is a decrease in the possibility to transform phosphorylase and to reduce efficiency of the transformed enzyme by uncoupling, this could explain the decrease in the rate of glycogen degradation with the subsequent increase of FFA oxidation observed during prolonged exercise.

B. Saltin—Are there any similarities in the glycogenolysis regulation in invertebrates, for example, flying insects and mammals?

G. Wegener—Yes, basically the regulation of glycolysis in insects' flight muscle seems to be the same; what is different is that we do not find any effect of citrate on the phosphofructokinase. Insects when flying change from carbohydrate to fat metabolism similarly to exercising mammals, and fructose-2, 6-diphosphate is probably involved in the regulation of phosphofructokinase activity. Other possible factors that can be of importance are AMP and ammonium. Thus, the insect flight muscles can be a good model for studying both the mechanisms activating glycolysis during maximal exercise and those responsible for changes in the rate of glycolysis when prolonged work has to be done.

E. Hultman—Fructose-2, 6-diphosphate is also active in humans, but there are only very few studies on its effect on glycolysis. Small changes in this compound in human muscles suggest species differences in regulation of glycolysis.

B. Saltin—Another aspect of the glycolytic rate is the fact that pyruvate production can exceed possibilities of its handling by mitochondria and leads to a gradual increase in blood lactate (LA) concentration long before the maximal oxygen uptake is reached (at 60-80% $\dot{V}O_2$max).

K. Sahlin—When it comes to the question why LA accumulation occurs before the whole aerobic capacity is utilized, it should be mentioned that lactic acid formation and also creatine phosphate degradation at the submaximal exercise have their consequences for aerobic metabolism because increases in ADP, inorganic phosphate, and NADH activate local respiration. At higher work loads, all these factors accelerate glycolysis in excess of what is needed for the oxidation purposes. The percentage of maximal oxygen uptake which can be utilized by muscles before fatigue develops depends on local factors, that is, muscle oxygen utilization capacity determined to a great extent by mitochondrial density and activity of oxidative enzymes.

P.D. Gollnick—I am not convinced that it is related to hypoxia, since you can shift the anaerobic threshold by modifying glycogen content in muscle.

K. Sahlin—Of course oxygen tension is not the only factor influencing the rate of glycolysis. There is no direct link between oxygen tension and glycolysis. The latter is more directly related to the increases in ADP and P_i.

B. Saltin—As you can see, the problem of anaerobic threshold contains many controversies concerning its basic mechanism. Whatever the mechanism of LA accumulation, the threshold has proven to have an extremely high prognostic value in endurance-type sport events lasting longer than a few minutes.

Another unsolved problem, mentioned already during the Symposium, is why the endurance capacity of the elite athletes has been constantly increasing and will probably continue to increase in spite of the fact that cardiac volume and maximum oxygen uptake has not changed in comparison with the values reported within the last 50 years.

P.D. Gollnick—The most pronounced training effect so far described is an increase in muscle mitochondrial content, which can be easily doubled. This adaptation correlates well in longitudinal training studies with the improved endurance capacity. The important aspect of it is that it results in the most effective use of substrates available for muscles. The largest energy reserve of the body is certainly fat (about 100,000 Kcal in normal men). The problem, however, is the amount of carbohydrates available for muscles, which is critical, especially when they are used for lactate production. In addition, the central nervous system of humans requires above 100 g of glucose daily, so when blood glucose level becomes low as a result of exercise, then performance can be severely impaired. A training-induced increase in the density of mitochondria leads to the most effective use of all energy substrates available, especially glycogen. Some world class long-distance runners reach 80 to 90% of their aerobic capacity before they start to accumulate any appreciable amounts of lactate, thereby using oxidative processes to the greatest advantage.

B. Saltin—Since the most efficient use of energy substrates determines to a great extent exercise performance, mobilization of extramuscular substrates is of importance for prolonged exercise. Dr. Nazar promised to present some current opinions on this topic.

K. Nazar—During exercise it is of importance to maintain an optimal proportion of carbohydrate to fat utilization for a certain task. The best strategy is to use enough carbohydrates to ensure the high rate of energy generation, but without exhausting their body stores and subsequent deprivation of the central nervous system of glucose. Contribution of carbohydrates and lipids to exercise metabolism depends on the intracellular mechanisms already discussed and on the extramuscular substrate availability. The latter is related to the action of hormones controlling glucose mobilization from the liver and FFA from adipose tissue. After training most hormonal responses to exercise are attenuated, but at the same time tissue sensitivity to many hormones increases. As an end result, the effects of hormones on substrate utilization seem to be the same before and after training.

But, of course, the strategy of substrate mobilization can be modified by nutritional factors. It is possible, for example, to increase body carbohydrate stores by a carbohydrate-rich diet, or by giving glucose or a carbohydrate-rich meal before or during exercise. However, the latter procedure changes the hormonal status, increasing insulin secretion. One should be aware that this, in turn, can inhibit fat mobilization, so it may not be beneficial for a long performance, for example, a marathon run. On the other hand, it may be of some value in case of exercise of short duration promoting high carbohydrate utilization and enabling the higher power output. Interactions between hormonal effects, changes in substrate availability, and intramuscular mechanisms controlling fuel utilization are important areas for further studies.

B. Saltin—It seems to us that we possess large basic knowledge about adaptation to exercise and we apply it in practice. What we do not know, however, is, what is the stimulus triggering these adaptations? This problem seems to me a challenge for physiologists working in the field of exercise physiology. Today, new possibilities exist to study this at the level of transcription and translation in muscle cells, obtained by biopsies from human muscles. What is the potential of such an approach and how close are we to unraveling the mechanism of the events regulating protein synthesis?

P.D. Gollnick—The area of exercise physiology and biochemistry, like all others, has to constantly look to the future. We now have a rather complete description of training adaptations and are beginning to understand what their significance is to performance. Another important area is that of muscular atrophy produced by a variety of conditions.

Clearly, the future lies in the identification of the cellular mechanisms that control the adaptive responses. In order to make substantial progress in these areas, it will be necessary to use the new methods of cellular and molecular biology to establish where and how protein synthesis is controlled. The ultimate questions that will be asked in this area are, what are the factor or factors that induce changes and how are they sensed at the level of the genes that control protein synthesis? As a final comment, I would make a plea; those individuals who work on a molecular or subcellular level should constantly try to relate their findings to total body function.

Reference

Milner-Brown, H.S., Stein, R.B., & Lee, R.G. (1975). Synchronization of human motor units: Possible role of exercise in supraspinal reflexes. *Electroencephalography in Clinical Neurophysiology, 38*, 245-254.